Annual of
Lymphoid Malignancies

Annual of Lymphoid Malignancies

Edited by

Franco Cavalli MD FRCP
Director, Oncology Institute of Southern Switzerland
Ospedale San Giovanni
Bellinzona, Switzerland

James O Armitage MD
Dean of the School of Medicine
Professor, Department of Internal Medicine
University of Nebraska Medical Center
Omaha, NE, USA

Dan L Longo MD FACP
Scientific Director
National Institute on Aging
National Institutes of Health
Baltimore, MD, USA

MARTIN DUNITZ

© Martin Dunitz Ltd 2001

First published in the United Kingdom in 2001 by
Martin Dunitz Ltd
The Livery House
7–9 Pratt Street
London NW1 0AE

Tel: +44-(0)20-7482-2202
Fax: +44-(0)20-7267-0159
E-mail: info.dunitz@tandf.co.uk
Website: http://www.dunitz.co.uk

A CIP catalogue record for this book is available from the British Library

ISBN 1-84184-000-9

Distributed in the United States by:
Blackwell Science Inc.
Commerce Place, 350 Main Street
Malden, MA 02148, USA
Tel: 1-800-215-1000

Distributed in Canada by:
Login Brothers Book Company
324 Salteaux Cresent
Winnipeg, Manitoba R3J 3T2
Canada
Tel: 1-204-224-4068

Distributed in Brazil by:
Ernesto Reichmann Distribuidora de Livros, Ltda
Rua Coronel Marques 335, Tatuape 03440-000
Sao Paulo,
Brazil

Composition by Wearset, Boldon, Tyne and Wear.
Printed and bound in Great Britain by Biddles Ltd. Guildford and King's Lynn.

Contents

Preface

This is the first of a series of annual reviews that will aim to summarize the most important and exciting progress that has been achieved during the preceding year in the field of malignant lymphomas, through a comprehensive review of the literature and trial data.

Lymphoid malignancies are of key importance for haemato-oncologists, since they represent a group of diseases whose incidence has doubled in the last fifteen years. However, important progress has been achieved in the therapy of these diseases, largely as a result of the extensive growth of knowledge in the biologic field, and therefore it can be claimed that every year the cure rate is improving, although not as quickly as we would wish to see. Nevertheless, there is a real hope in the next few years that therapeutic outcomes will dramatically improve.

As a result of these rapid changes, even specialists in this field have difficulty keeping in touch with the latest developments. The main aim of this series is therefore to enable not only haemato-oncologists, but also biologists interested in lymphomas, to see at a glance how the field is developing. We hope that this book will go some way to achieving this ambitious goal.

Franco Cavalli
James O Armitage
Dan L Longo

Contributors

James O Armitage, MD
Department of Internal Medicine
University of Nebraska Medical
Center
600 South 42nd Street
Omaha, NE 68109-3332
USA

Daniele Bernardi, MD
Division of Medical Oncology A
National Cancer Institute
Via Pedemontana Occ.le 12
I-33081 Aviano (PN)
Italy

Francesco Bertoni, MD
Department of Experimental
Haematology
St Bartholomew's & the Royal
London Hospitals
School of Medicine & Dentistry
Turner Street
London E1 2AD
UK

Franco Cavalli, MD
Oncology Institute of Southern
Switzerland
Ospedale San Giovanni
CH-6500 Bellinzona
Switzerland

Bertrand Coiffier, MD
Service d'Hématologie Clinique
Pavillion Marcel Bérard 1F
Centre Hospitalier Lyon-Sud
F-69495 Pierre-Bénite Cedex
France

Annarita Conconi, MD
Division of Medical Oncology
Oncology Institute of Southern
Switzerland
Ospedale San Giovanni
CH-6500 Bellinzona
Switzerland

Dennis Cooper, MD
Department of Internal Medicine
Section of Medical Oncology
Yale University School of Medicine
333 Cedar Street
New Haven, CT 06520-8032
USA

**Finbarr Cotter, PhD, FRCP,
FRCPath**
Department of Experimental
Haematology
St Bartholomew's & the Royal
London Hospitals
School of Medicine & Dentistry
Turner Street
London E1 2AD
UK

Martin Dreyling, MD
Klinikum Grosshadern
Medizinische Klinik III
Marchioninistrasse 15
D-81377 Munich
Germany

Richard I Fisher, MD
Cardinal Bernardin Cancer Center
Loyola University Chicago
2160 South First Avenue
Maywood, IL 60153
USA

John E Godwin, MD, MS
Division of Hematology/Oncology
Loyola University Chicago
2160 South First Avenue
Maywood, IL 60153
USA

Gösta Gahrton, MD
Department of Medicine
Karolinska Institutet
Huddinge University Hospital
S-14186 Stockholm
Sweden

Wolfgang Hiddemann, MD, PhD
Klinikum Grosshadern
Medizinische Klinik III
Marchioninistrasse 15
D-81377 Munich
Germany

Sandra J Horning, MD
Division of Oncology
Stanford University Medical Center
1000 Welch Road, Suite 202
Palo Alto, CA 94304-5756
USA

Dan L Longo MD FACP
National Institute on Aging
National Institutes of Health
Gerontology Research Center
4940 Eastern Avenue
Baltimore, MD 21224-2780
USA

Jennifer B Lucas, MD
Oncology Fellowship Training
Program
Division of Oncology
Stanford University Medical Center
1000 Welch Road, Suite 202
Palo Alto, CA 94304-5756
USA

Ian Magrath, MD
INCTR
Institut Pasteur
Rue Engeland 642
B-1180 Brussels
Belgium

Paul N Mainwaring, MD
Department of Oncology
St Thomas' Hospital
Lambeth Palace Road
London SE5 7EH
UK

Angela Manns, MD, MPH
Genetic Epidemiology Branch
Division of Cancer Epidemiology and
Genetics
National Cancer Institute
6120 Executive Blvd.
Rockville, MD 20852
USA

Tanja Meyer, MD
Klinikum Grosshadern
Medizinische Klinik III
Marchioninstrasse 15
D-81377 Munich
Germany

Emilio Montserrat, MD
Department of Hematology
Institute of Hematology & Oncology
Hospital Clinic
University of Barcelona
Villarroel, 170
E-08036 Barcelona
Spain

Stuart Seropian, MD
Department of Internal Medicine
Section of Medical Oncology
Yale University School of Medicine
333 Cedar Street
New Haven, CT 06520-8032
USA

Maria Sgambati, MD
Genetic Epidemiology Branch
Division of Cancer Epidemiology and
Genetics
National Cancer Institute
6120 Executive Blvd.
Rockville, MD 20852
USA

Michele Spina, MD
Division of Medical Oncology A
National Cancer Institute
Via Pedemontana Occ.le 12
I-33081 Aviano (PN)
Italy

Adrian R Timothy, MD, MB, FRCP, FRCR
Clinical Oncology
St Thomas' Hospital
Lambeth Palace Road
London SE1 7EH
UK

Umberto Tirelli, MD
Division of Medical Oncology A
National Cancer Institute
Via Pedemontana Occ.le 12
I-33081 Aviano (PN)
Italy

Emanuele Zucca, MD
Division of Medical Oncology
Oncology Institute of Southern
Switzerland
Ospedale San Giovanni
CH-6500 Bellinzona
Switzerland

1
Epidemiology and pathogenesis of lymphoid malignancies

Angela Manns, Maria Sgambati

INTRODUCTION

Lymphoid malignancies constitute approximately 7% of total new cancer cases reported annually in the USA. A total of 84 000 new lymphoid cancers are estimated from surveillance data for the year 2000.[1] These neoplasms originate from the malignant transformation of bone marrow stem-cell-derived T or B lymphocytes. Normally these lymphocytes play an important physiologic role in the host's immune response to pathogens and foreign antigens. Through unknown mechanisms, the functional dysregulation of these cells results in neoplastic change, and uncontrolled growth and proliferation. The major adult lymphoid neoplasms include non-Hodgkin's lymphoma (NHL), chronic lymphocytic leukemia (CLL), Hodgkin's disease (HD), and multiple myeloma (MM). Each of these malignancies represents a distinct entity derived from lymphoid cells at various stages of maturation.

TRENDS IN INCIDENCE AND MORTALITY RATES (1973–1997)

Temporal trends in the incidence rates (new cases diagnosed per year per 100 000) and mortality rates of lymphoid malignancies over the past 24 years (1973–1997), as reported by the Surveillance Epidemiology and End Results Program (SEER),[2] are shown for males and females in Figure 1.1. NHLs represent the largest proportion of lymphoid neoplasms. Increasing incidence and mortality rates have been observed among NHLs in the USA, Europe, and elsewhere.[3] The reasons for the increase in incidence among both sexes and all races are not known. Between 1973 and 1997, the incidence rate for males changed from 10 to 19.2 per 100 000, with a peak rate of 20.7 in 1995. The incidence rate for females ranged from 7.4 to 13 per 100 000, the highest reported rates being in 1994 and 1997. Mortality rates have also increased, with rates for males increasing from 5.8 to 8.7 per 100 000 and for females from 3.9 to 5.7 per 100 000. Five-year relative survival rates have remained at

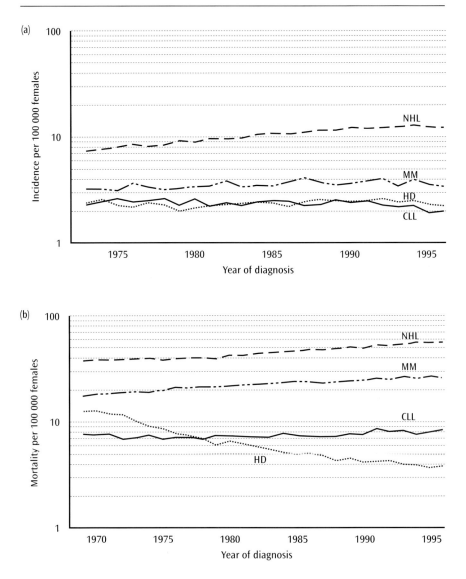

(a)

Incidence per 100 000 females

NHL

MM

HD

CLL

Year of diagnosis

(b)

Mortality per 100 000 females

NHL

MM

CLL

HD

Year of diagnosis

about 50% for the 24-year period. The small improvement in rates may be due to a disproportionate increase in cases among older persons (>65 years) and the resulting lack of optimal treatment. Because of the high frequency of co-morbid medical conditions at the time of NHL diagnosis in the elderly, chemotherapy is offered less often.[4,5]

The other lymphoid neoplasms have lower incidences and varying mortality rates compared with NHLs (Figure 1.1 and Table 1.1). The incidence rates in particular for CLL and HD have had a relatively stable trend over time (Table 1.1). CLL and HD have similar incidence rates, and these rates have shown a

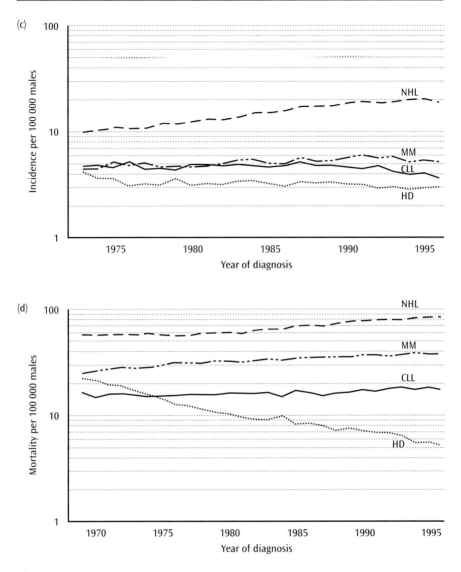

Figure 1.1

Time trends of incidence rates (a, c) and mortality rates (b, d) for lymphoid malignancies among females (a, b) and males (c, d) in the USA. Data are from SEER,[2] based on rates (per 100 000 on a log scale) age-adjusted to the 1970 US standard population. NHL, non-Hodgkin's lymphoma; MM, multiple myeloma; CLL, chronic lymphocytic leukemia; HD, Hodgkin's disease.

Table 1.1 Trends in incidence, mortality and five-year survival rates for lymphoid malignancies

	Non-Hodgkin's lymphoma	Multiple myeloma	Hodgkin's disease	Chronic lymphocytic leukemia
Incidence (per 100 000)				
1973	10	3.8	3.3	3.4
1997	19.2	4.4	2.7	2.6
Mortality (per 100 000)				
1973	5.8	2.3	1.3	1.1
1997	8.7	3.1	0.4	1.2
Five-year relative survival rate (%)				
1974–1976	47.2	24.5	71.2	68.5
1989–1996	51.6	28.5	82.1	71.4

decrease over the last 24 years. The CLL incidence rate changed from 3.4 to 2.6 per 100 000, with a peak of 3.6 in 1976 and 1987. Mortality rates for CLL remained stable, with changes from 1.1 to 1.2 per 100 000. Five-year relative survival rates have improved slightly from 68.5% to 71.4%, a statistically significant difference. No major impact of changes in therapy have been observed.

Incidence rates for HD changed from 3.3 to 2.7 per 100 000; this was a significant decline in the rates, observed particularly for males. The HD mortality rate changed from 1.3 to 0.4 per 100 000, which is a significant decline. The most significant decline was observed in the 1970s, particularly from 1973 to 1979. These changes were temporally related to the introduction of the MOPP regimen (mechlorethamine, vincristine, prednisone, and procarbazine). The decline in mortality has continued, with a fall (albeit not as dramatic) also being observed between 1979 and 1997. Five-year relative survival rates have improved significantly from 71.2% (1974–1976) to 82.1% (1989–1996).

MM has a slightly higher incidence rate than HD and CLL. The rates changed from 3.8 to 4.4 per 100 000, with a peak of 4.9 in 1991 in the USA. The most striking feature of this disease is the difference in incidence for Blacks compared with Whites and other racial groups. Incidence rates for Blacks changed from 9.7 to 8.6 per 100 000, with a peak of 11 in 1983. Mortality rates for MM have also shown a significant increase. Rates have changed from 2.3 to 3.1 per 100 000, with a significant increase being observed between 1973 and 1995. In more recent years (1995–1997), a decline in mortality of about 1% has been evident for males but not females. Females showed a significant 1–2% increase between 1973 and 1997. The five-year relative survival is lower for MM than for any other lymphoid malignancy. This may partly be due to the older median age at diagnosis and the resulting poorer prognosis for elderly patients that have also been observed for the NHLs. Alternatively, it suggests that MM is highly unresponsive to available chemotherapeutic regimens. The five-year relative survival rate has shown a small but significant increase from 24.5% to 28.5%.

RISK FACTORS ASSOCIATED WITH LYMPHOID MALIGNANCIES

To provide clues to the etiology and provide an explanation for the varying patterns of lymphoid malignancy rates observed, the following sections will review the potential risk factors reported in the literature in 1999. The primary focus will be on NHL and CLL. Selected references for further reading on MM and HD are provided at the end of the numbered reference list.

NON-HODGKIN'S LYMPHOMA

Background/demographics

NHLs are one of the most important cancers, with a largely unexplained increase in incidence. For the year 2000, an estimated 54 900 cases of NHL are predicted.[2] The incidence of NHL increases markedly with age at diagnosis, with rates of 9/100 000 for cases under age 65 years, compared with 76/100 000 for those diagnosed over age 65 years (Figure 1.2).[6] Males have an

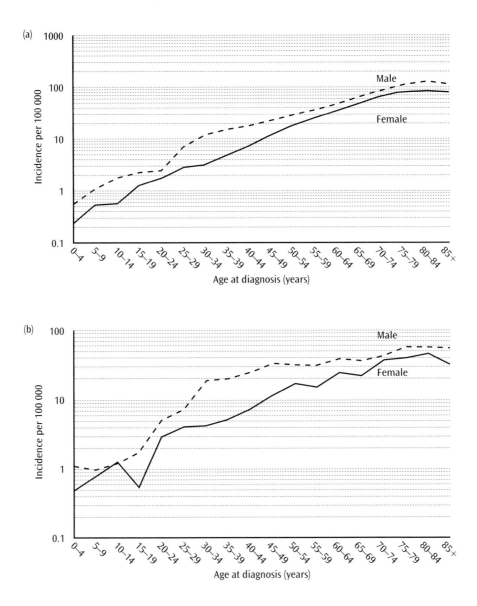

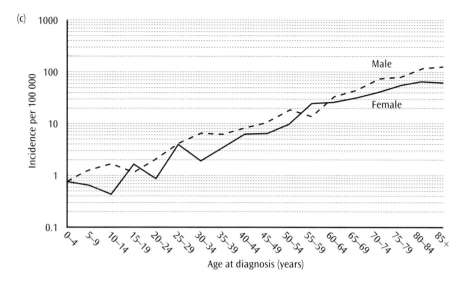

Figure 1.2

Age-, sex-, and race-specific incidence rates for non-Hodgkin's lymphoma from SEER[6] (1992–1996): (a) Whites; (b) Blacks; (c) other races (including Asian/Pacific Islander, Native American, and Hispanic).

incidence nearly 1.5- to 2-fold higher than females. Whites have rates of 16/100 000, which are slightly higher than the rates for Blacks of 13/100 000. These age-, sex-, and race-specific differences may provide useful etiologic clues.

The variation in incidence with age may suggest that an exposure or risk is inherent to the aging process or requires a large cumulative dose before NHL develops. The gender-specific difference in rates could reflect risk from exposures such as occupation or occupation-related environmental factors that differ by sex. The gender differences could also be related to sex-linked genes such as the Xq28 region, a hypothesis recently suggested by Vineis et al.[7] The X-linked locus for glucose-6-phosphate dehydrogenase (G6PD) is located in the region, and a fivefold excess of NHL has been identified in a cohort of G6PD-deficient men.

Racial/ethnic disparities suggest differences either in genetic susceptibility or in environment; the latter differences may be influenced by lifestyle and related to factors such as socioeconomic status. Few studies have been conducted that compare risk factors for NHL between racial/ethnic groups. Interestingly, although increases in incidence rates are widespread worldwide, there are still areas with relatively low incidence rates, supporting a geographic variability in risk. Population heterogeneity reflects differences in possible etiologic factors, and is further underscored by geographic variation in the occurrence of histologic subtypes. A recent report from Japan revealed that the classification of B-cell NHL according to the Revised European American Lymphoma (REAL) classification in that country demonstrated differences in the frequency of subtypes compared with Western countries.[8] Diffuse large B-cell lymphomas were more frequent (58.8% versus 31%) and follicular lymphomas less frequent (12% versus 22%) in Japan compared with Western countries.

Histologic classification

NHLs constitute a heterogeneous group of cancers that differ in their biologic behavior, clinical characteristics, and histologic types. The REAL classification was introduced in 1994 with the aim to more accurately define and categorize lymphoid malignancies. This classification scheme considered histopathology, immunophenotype, genetic, and clinical features. After several years experience with the REAL classification, the World Health Organization (WHO) assembled a team of experts to further refine the classification and broaden the consensus. An important report by the WHO group answered some controversial questions arising in the REAL classification, and provided several improvements of clinical relevance.[9] Key findings pertinent to the lymphoid malignancies were as follows:

1. Acute lymphoblastic leukemias (ALL) and lymphoblastic lymphomas are a single disease with different clinical presentations.
2. B-cell chronic lymphocytic leukemia (B-CLL) and B-cell small lymphocytic lymphoma are a single disease at different stages.
3. The nomenclature for follicle center lymphoma was changed to follicular lymphoma, and specific guidelines for grading and identifying diffuse areas were recommended because of their prognostic significance.
4. The term 'extranodal marginal zone B-cell lymphoma of MALT' is only to be applied to lymphoma composed mostly of small cells.
5. Nodal and splenic marginal zone lymphomas are distinct diseases.
6. Clinical syndromes such as mycosis fungoides are essential to the definition of peripheral T/NK-cell neoplasms.
7. Cutaneous anaplastic large cell lymphoma (ALCL) and systemic ALCL are probably distinct entities.
8. Clinical groupings of lymphoid malignancies similar to those in the Working Formulation classification are not necessary.

Factors influencing immunity – non-infectious and infectious agents

Perturbations of normal immunologic function are important in lymphoma-genesis. Several mechanisms have been proposed to be implicated in this process, and have recently been reviewed.[10,11] During the course of the normal immune response, antigenic stimulation resulting in B-cell proliferation may result in genetic instability.[11] The genetic instability associated with lymphoid malignancies generally results in chromosomal translocations involving the antigen receptor loci. The common translocations associated with B-cell lymphoid malignancies include c-MYC (t(8;14), t(2;8) and t(8;22) in Burkitt's lymphoma), BCL2 (t(14;18) in follicular lymphoma), BCL1 (t(11;14) in mantle cell lymphoma), BCL6 (t(3;14) in large cell lymphoma), and BCL3 (t(14;19) in B-CLL). These translocations initiate the oncogenic pathway. Other genetic events and abnormalities in the repair of DNA damage are also required.

Important pathogenic clues can be obtained through the study of hereditary immunodeficiency syndromes where the genetic defects associated with immunodeficiency are known. For example, ataxia telangiectasia (AT) is an autosomal recessive disorder characterized by cerebellar ataxia, telangiectasias on sun-exposed surfaces, hypersensitivity to ionizing radiation, and defects in cellular and humoral immunity.[10,11] AT occurs primarily in children (with a median age at diagnosis of 8.5 years), with a male predominance. The gene associated with AT is called ATM (mutated in ataxia telangiectasia) and is located at 11q22–23. The ATM protein plays a signaling role that is important in receiving information from molecules that detect DNA damage. The cells of AT patients have a heightened sensitivity to agents that induce double-strand DNA breaks, and manifest abnormal cell cycle regulation in response to DNA damage. Interestingly, the chromosomal abnormalities in AT involve predominantly T lymphocytes. Thirty-eight percent of AT patients develop cancers, and 85% of these are lymphoid neoplasms, predominantly of T-cell origin.

Several other conditions and exposures associated with immune suppression are also of interest. Organ transplant recipients receiving immunosuppressive therapy are at increased risk for NHL and other malignancies.[10] NHLs in this setting are usually aggressive, high-grade, and extranodal, and since transplant recipients have impaired host defenses against Epstein–Barr virus (EBV), most are EBV-positive. Primary effusion lymphoma, the newly described entity sometimes associated with human herpesvirus type 8/Kaposi's sarcoma-associated herpesvirus (HHV8/KSHV), has recently been reported after heart transplantation.[12]

Allogeneic blood transfusions have been hypothesized to have immunosuppressive potential. Additionally, transfusions may harbor infectious agents not routinely screened, such as EBV, cytomegalovirus (CMV), and HHV8. Two case–control studies evaluated whether blood transfusion recipients have an increased risk for the development of NHL.[13,14] One study showed no association with a history of transfusion and risk for NHL, irrespective of NHL histologic grade.[13] The second study stratified on the temporal relationship of transfusion to development of NHL. A significantly increased risk was identified among cases having a transfusion within the three months prior to diagnosis; however, no association was seen if transfusion had been given more than three months before diagnosis. Thus, the authors concluded that this finding most likely represented treatment of early disease. Conflicting results have been reported in the literature. Most of the previous studies showing a positive association have been cohort study designs.[13,14]

A number of reports have explored the possible link between various infectious agents and the development of NHL. These agents infect T or B cells, resulting in an immune response that may provoke chronic antigenic stimulation and cellular proliferation or cause immune suppression. Human immunodeficiency virus (HIV) infection has been one of the most frequently studied.[15-19] The topic of greatest interest was investigation of the effect of antiretroviral therapy on trends of NHL and other malignant outcomes. The general consensus was that the incidence of malignancy was decreasing for Kaposi's sarcoma and also some subtypes of NHL. One report showed that the incidence of primary brain lymphoma significantly decreased over a three-year period, whereas no significant changes were seen for immunoblastic lymphomas, Burkitt's lymphoma, other NHLs, or HD.[20] Another pertinent report examined the *CCR5* chemokine receptor gene in relation to risk for HIV-related NHL.[21] A mutation in this gene prevents expression of the receptor on cell surfaces and protects against HIV infection and disease progression. The study found a three-fold lower risk for NHL among individuals heterozygous for *CCR5-Δ32*. Based on these reports, a risk profile for NHL susceptibility can be determined among HIV carriers by identifying *CCR5* gene status, and the use of antiretroviral therapy can prevent the development of NHL.

Among other viruses studied, EBV, commonly associated with B-cell NHL, was also frequently (19/32(59%)) detected in various T-cell NHLs by in situ hybridization with an RNA probe specific to EBV-specific nuclear antigen 1 (EBNA-1).[22] In addition, a novel EBV-like virus has been reported in association with mycosis fungoides.[23] Several small seroprevalence studies found no association between hepatitis C virus (HCV) and B-cell NHL,[24,25] although another small cross-sectional study found the prevalence of HCV to be significantly more frequent in NHLs with mixed cryoglobulinemia.[26]

Autoimmune conditions have been implicated as a possible risk factor for NHLs. Frequently reported conditions associated with NHL include rheumatoid arthritis, Sjögren's syndrome, and celiac disease.[27-29] The mechanism of NHL pathogenesis may be associated with immune-related features of these disorders that lead to chronic antigenic stimulation and lymphocyte proliferation. In a report of patients with celiac disease[27] – a chronic disorder characterized by small bowel villous atrophy that impairs nutrient absorption – B-cell NHLs of the stomach were common, suggesting that local antigen stimulus probably preceded development of NHL.

Another interesting report evaluated artificial joint implants as a possible risk factor for various cancers, including NHL.[30] Many reports in the literature have examined this question in the context of breast implants; however, none have evaluated risk in patients with artificial joint implants, despite their widespread use. The study by Fryzek et al[30] found no increased risk of NHL or other cancers in patients with artificial joints, except for those also with a diagnosis of rheumatoid arthritis (RA). There was a fivefold increase in the incidence of NHL among patients with RA. A second report[29] attempted to elucidate the possible mechanisms for the development of NHL in RA patients.

These authors compared patients with NHL and RA with patients with NHL and no RA, but found no significant differences in the occurrence of lymphoproliferative disorders containing EBV (2%), site of NHL presentation (primarily extranodal), grade (predominantly low and intermediate), or immunophenotype (predominantly B-cell NHL). However, marginal zone lymphomas (mucosa-associated lymphoid tissue (MALT) lymphomas) were more common among patients with NHL and RA. MALT lymphomas appear to be related to chronic antigenic stimulation and are frequently associated with *Helicobacter pylori*.[31–33] Further research is required to fully understand these possible relationships.

Personal and lifestyle factors

Certain personal traits may characterize host genetic background, while various lifestyle or behavioural factors may be indicative of environmental exposures that are important determinants of risk. The most substantive report examining these factors during 1999 was a large case–control study performed by Holly et al.[34] This study collected data from 1281 cases and 2095 controls from the San Francisco Bay area of California. An extensive face-to-face interview was conducted with detailed questions about personal, family, medical (including medication and immunizations), and job and travel history. The most intriguing findings revealed a reduced risk of NHL associated with a history of various allergies and potential immune system stimuli such as an increase in the number of bee and wasp stings and vaccinations. The authors proposed that the positive effects of immune stimulation were associated with a persistent capacity for B-cell differentiation and a decrease in accumulation of B cells or enhanced apoptosis. Significant factors associated with an increased risk of NHL for both males and females included a history of lymphoma in the immediate family, which conferred a two- to three-fold excess, the use of ulcer medications (cimetidine and others), and increased body mass index (BMI = weight [kg]/height [m^2]). The increase in risk with use of ulcer medication could be a surrogate marker for people who are also infected with *Helicobacter pylori*. The increased risk associated with BMI may be due to dietary factors.

An important analysis conducted in the Nurse's Health Study examined dietary fat and protein in relation to risk of NHL among women.[35] Animal studies have shown that fat, particularly *n*-6 polyunsaturated fatty acids, can be immune-suppressive. However, this has not been demonstrated in humans. In this report, height greater than 62 inches (1.57 m) was associated with an increased risk of NHL, but increased BMI was not. *Trans* unsaturated fats significantly increased the risk of NHL; major sources of such fats include foods such as meats (beef, pork, lamb), and home-made pies and cakes. Broiled and barbecued meats appeared to confer greater risk than roasted, pan-fried, boiled, or stewed meats. Identification of adverse factors associated with increased meat consumption will need to be explored.

Other factors reported that merit further mention are an increased risk of

NHL in association with sunlight exposure (ultraviolet light dose) and various pesticides, including herbicides (2,4-dichlorophenoxyacetic acid) and fungicides.[36,37] Pesticide use is widespread in the occupational and residential setting. These exposures generate important hypotheses to be pursued, and are topics for future studies in the USA and elsewhere.

CHRONIC LYMPHOCYTIC LEUKEMIA

Background/demographics

As mentioned earlier, CLL and the NHL subtypes of small lymphocytic lymphomas represent different stages of the same disease.[9] Small lymphocytic lymphomas represent about 8% of the total NHLs reported to SEER.[2] CLL represents 30% of leukemias, and has a similar incidence to acute myeloid leukemia but a greater incidence than acute lymphoblastic and chronic myeloid leukemias. In 2000, an estimated 8100 new cases of CLL will be diagnosed in the USA.[1] SEER Registry Data indicate that incidence rates are highest among white males (4.2/100 000) and lowest among other races (Figure 1.3). Ethnic variation in incidence rates is well documented in CLL. A study from Mexico[38] reported that, in contrast to other Western countries, CLL is the least frequent subtype of leukemia among Mexican mestizos (individuals with mixed European and Native American ancestry).

Similar to NHL, the incidence of CLL also increases markedly with age at diagnosis, with rates of 1.2/100 000 for cases under the age of 65 years, compared with 20/100 000 for those diagnosed over the age of 65. The major general topic of interest in CLL in 1999 was the increasing recognition of the

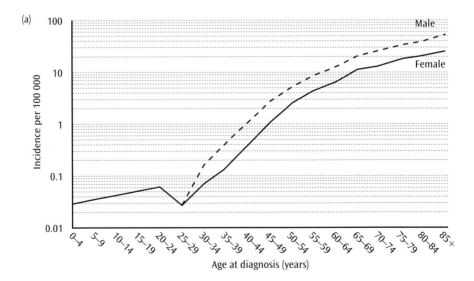

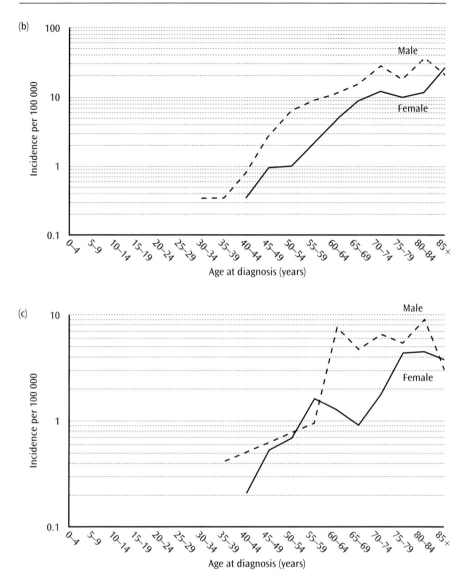

Figure 1.3

Age-, sex-, and race-specific incidence rates for chronic lymphocytic leukemia from SEER[6] (1992–1996): (a) Whites; (b) Blacks; (c) other races (including Asian/Pacific Islander, Native American, and Hispanic).

heterogeneity in CLL, challenging long-held beliefs that CLL is a benign disease of the elderly. Appreciation of this variability in disease behavior was noted on both a clinical and molecular level. In a single-institution study examining the effect of age at diagnosis on outcome, young CLL cases (55 years or younger) were found to have a higher risk of Richter's transformation when compared with older CLL cases (over 55 years).[39] Additionally, a different distribution of cause of death was seen among the younger cohort, and younger patients were more likely to die from CLL rather than other causes.[39] While overall survival was similar between the two groups, expected survival was more adversely affected in the younger cohort. Presence of active disease or a lymphocyte doubling time of less than 12 months identified a subgroup of the younger cohort with a worse prognosis.

Occupational and environmental exposures

Although there was no major epidemiological study on CLL alone in 1999, several reports did investigate the role of exposures in the development of cancer and lymphoproliferative disorders. In a report of a Swedish cohort study investigating occupational magnetic field exposure and cancer risk, no association was found with CLL.[40] An Italian case–control study of occupational and lifestyle exposure found small increases in CLL risk with smoking and the professions of hairdressing, textile work, and teaching; however, CLL was analyzed together with NHL and not as a separate category.[41] A study evaluating the risk of leukemia and radiation exposure among Japanese atomic bomb survivors, women treated for cervical cancer, and patients treated for ankylosing spondylitis found no evidence of increased risk of CLL among the latter two groups.[42] This confirms previous reports of no association between radiation and the development of CLL. A report investigating the role of sunlight exposure in lymphoma found no association with CLL.[36] A role for viruses in the etiology continues to be a subject of research interest. In a Japanese study, two out of seven CLL cases showed high levels of HHV6 by quantitative PCR–ELISA.[43]

Pathogenesis/prognostic indicators

With the acceleration in the development of techniques in molecular biology, the search for disease-associated biomarkers has become an area of intense interest. Novel prognostic indicators may help improve patient treatment and care, as well as leading to improved understanding of etiology and carcinogenesis in CLL. Several molecular and genetic events have been highlighted in CLL. Several reports of immunoglobulin (Ig) gene variability in CLL made the news in 1999. One of the more important findings was the association of unmutated versus mutated immunoglobulin variable gene rearrangements with clinical behavior in CLL, reinforcing the heterogeneity of the disease.[44] Individuals with unmutated Ig genes[44,45] and CD38 overexpression[45] had more aggressive disease and a poorer outcome as compared with individuals with mutated Ig genes and low CD38 expression.

There were several other reports of molecular abnormalities associated with CLL. Cyclin D1 overexpression (resulting from the t(11;14) translocation) was found in a subset of atypical CLL cases behaving more aggressively than typical CLL and with clinical features suggestive of MCL (mantle cell lymphoma).[46] Other studies confirmed previous reports of more advanced disease and a shorter overall survival with higher cell surface CD14 positivity[47] and the association of increased levels of β_2-microglobulin and soluble CD23 (sCD23) with a worse clinical outcome.[48]

The *ATM* gene mentioned earlier in association with NHL also remains an area of active investigation in CLL. As previously mentioned, the *ATM* gene is mutated in patients with ataxia telangiectasia; however, current data are mixed regarding its role in CLL. A report of linkage analysis for the *ATM* gene in familial CLL found no evidence for association;[49] however, the study may have lacked the power to find a link. However, another group found impaired ATM protein expression in 40% of cases and germline and tumor mutations in *ATM* in a smaller portion of cases.[50] The mechanism of *ATM* mutations in the pathogenesis is unknown; however, one possible mechanism is through expression of adhesion molecules on the surfaces of lymphocytes. CLL cells with an 11q deletion carried significantly lower levels of some cell surface adhesion molecules and lower expression of specific cell signaling receptors.[51]

FUTURE DIRECTIONS

The increasing incidence of NHL is perplexing, because much of it cannot be explained by the exposures and risks that are currently known. NHL is a heterogeneous disease, and an adjustment of our current approaches will be facilitated by implementation of the REAL/WHO classification. However, before this classification proves useful, changes in current practices of diagnosing NHL must take effect. A concerted effort must be made to conduct the necessary immunophenotyping that is required. Additional molecular characterization with new technology such as microarrays will also assist in defining NHL subtypes. The identification of new exposures can then be facilitated. For example, it is interesting that autoimmune conditions such as rheumatoid arthritis and celiac disease are associated with MALT lymphomas. What is the role of *Helicobacter pylori* in disease pathogenesis? Such insights provide clues to guide further epidemiologic investigations.

CLL and the NHL subtype of small lymphocytic lymphomas are the same disease at different stages. Comparative studies of these similar disease entities and others may provide useful information about potential risk factors. Hopefully, the next few years will bring progress in understanding the etiology of CLL and NHL. Molecular biology and genetic mapping efforts will help delineate candidate genes. As understanding of the heterogeneity of the disease increases, future studies will focus on novel prognostic factors that may also serve as therapeutic targets. Attempts to elucidate environmental factors will be enhanced by integration with molecular biomarker data. Similar approaches should also be undertaken to further our understanding of Hodgkin's disease and multiple myeloma.

REFERENCES

1. *Cancer Facts and Figures 2000.* Atlanta, GA: American Cancer Society, 2000: 4–5.

2. SEER*Stat Software (SEER Cancer Incidence Public-Use Database, 1973–1997). Bethesda, MD: National Cancer Institute, 2000.

3. Cartwright R, Brincker H, Carli PM et al, The rise in incidence of lymphomas in Europe 1985–1992. *Eur J Cancer* 1999; **35**: 627–33.

4. Peters FPJ, Haaft MA Ten, Schouten HC, Intermediate and high grade non Hodgkin's lymphoma in the elderly. *Leuk Lymphoma* 1999; **33**: 243–52.

5. Van Spronsen DJ, Janssen-Heijnen MLG, Breed WPM, Coebergh JWW, Prevalence of co-morbidity and its relationship to treatment among unselected patients with Hodgkin's disease and non-Hodgkin's lymphoma, 1993–1996. *Ann Hematol* 1999; **78**: 315–19.

6. Ries LAG, Kosary CL, Hankey BF et al (eds), *SEER Cancer Statistics Review, 1973–1996.* Bethesda, MD: National Cancer Institute, NIH Publication 99-2789, 1999.

7. Vineis P, Masala G, Costantini AS and the Working Group for the Epidemiology of Hematolymphopoietic Malignancies in Italy, Does a gene in the Xq28 region increase the risk of non-Hodgkin's lymphomas? *Ann Oncol* 1999; **10**: 471–3.

8. Ohshima K, Suzumiya J, Sato K et al, B-cell lymphoma of 708 cases in Japan: incidence rates and clinical prognosis according to the REAL classification. *Cancer Lett* 1999; **135**: 73–81.

9. Harris NL, Jaffe ES, Diebold J et al, World Health Organization classification of neoplastic diseases of the hematopoietic and lymphoid tissues: report of the Clinical Advisory Committee meeting – Airlie House, Virginia, November 1997. *J Clin Oncol* 1999; **17**: 3835–49.

10. Mueller N, Overview of the epidemiology of malignancy in immune deficiency. *J Acquir Immune Defic Syndr* 1999; **21**: S5–10.

11. Vanasse GJ, Concannon P, Willerford DM, Regulated genomic instability and neoplasia in the lymphoid lineage. *Blood* 1999; **94**: 3997–4010.

12. Dotti G, Fiocchi R, Motta T et al, Primary effusion lymphoma after heart transplantation: a new entity associated with human herpesvirus-8. *Leukemia* 1999; **13**: 664–70.

13. Maguire-Boston EK, Suman V, Jacobsen SJ et al, Blood transfusion and risk of non-Hodgkin's lymphoma. *Am J Epidemiol* 1999; **149**: 1113–18.

14. Tavani A, Soler M, LaVecchia C, Franceschi S, Blood transfusions and the risk of intermediate- or high-grade non-Hodgkin's lymphoma. *J Natl Cancer Inst* 1999; **91**: 1332–3.

15. Sparano JA, Anand K, Desai J et al, Effect of highly active antiretroviral therapy on the incidence of HIV-associated malignancies at an Urban Medical Center. *J Acquir Immune Defic Syndr* 1999; **21**: S18–22.

16. Buchbinder SP, Holmberg SD, Scheer S et al, Combination antiretroviral therapy and incidence of AIDS-related malignancies. *J Acquir Immune Defic Syndr* 1999; **21**: S23–6.

17. Grulich AE, AIDS-associated non-Hodgkin's lymphoma in the era of highly active antiretroviral therapy. *J Acquir Immune Defic Syndr* 1999; **21**: S27–30.

18. Rabkin CS, Testa MA, Huang J, Von Roenn JH, Kaposi's sarcoma and non-Hodgkin's lymphoma incidence trends in AIDS clinical trial group study participants. *J Acquir Immun Defic Syndr* 1999; **21**: S31–3.

19. Jacobson LP, Yamashita TE, Detels R et al, for the Multicenter AIDS Cohort Study, Impact of potent antiretroviral therapy on the incidence of Kaposi's sarcoma and non-Hodgkin's lymphomas among HIV-1 infected individuals. *J Acquir Immune Defic Syndr* 1999; **21**: S34–41.

20. Jones JL, Hanson DL, Dworkin MS et

al, and the Adult/Adolescent Spectrum of HIV Disease Project Group, Effect of antiretroviral therapy on recent trends in selected cancers among HIV-infected persons. *J Acquir Immune Defic Syndr* 1999; **21**: S11–17.

21. Dean M, Jacobson LP, McFarlane G et al, Reduced risk of AIDS lymphoma in individuals heterozygous for the CCR5-Δ32 mutation. *Cancer Res* 1999; **59**: 3561–4.

22. Yamamoto T, Nakamura Y, Kishimoto K et al, Epstein–Barr virus (EBV)-infected cells were frequently but dispersely detected in T-cell lymphomas of various types by in situ hybridization with an RNA probe specific to EBV-specific nuclear antigen 1. *Virus Res* 1999; **65**: 43–55.

23. Rivadeneira ED, Ferrari MG, Jarrett RF et al, A novel Epstein–Barr virus-like virus, HV_MNE, in a *Macaca nemestrina* with mycosis fungoides. *Blood* 1999; **94**: 2090–101.

24. Shariff S, Yoshida EM, Gascoyne RD et al, Hepatitis C infection and B-cell non-Hodgkin's lymphoma in British Columbia: a cross-sectional analysis. *Ann Oncol* 1999; **10**: 961–4.

25. Collier JD, Zanke B, Moore M et al, No association between hepatitis C and B-cell lymphoma. *Hepatology* 1999; **29**: 1259–61.

26. Domingo JM, Romero S, Moreno JA et al, Hepatitis C virus infection and mixed cryoglobulinemia in patients with lymphoproliferative diseases. *Hematologica* 1999; **84**: 94–6.

27. Davidson BKS, Kelly CA, Griffiths ID, Primary Sjögren's syndrome in the north east of England: a long-term follow-up study. *Rheumatology* 1999; **38**: 245–53.

28. Cottone M, Termini A, Oliva L et al, Mortality and causes of death in celiac disease in a Mediterranean area. *Dig Dis Sci* 1999; **44**: 2538–47.

29. Kamel OW, Holly EA, van de Run M et al, A population based, case control study of non-Hodgkin's lymphoma in patients with rheumatoid arthritis. *J Rheumatol* 1999; **26**: 1676–80.

30. Fryzek JP, Mellemkjaer L, McLaughlin JK et al, Cancer risk among patients with finger and hand joint and temporo-mandibular joint prostheses in Denmark. *Int J Cancer* 1999; **81**: 723–5.

31. Au WY, Gascoyne RD, Le N et al, Incidence of second neoplasms in patients with MALT lymphoma: no increase in risk above the background population. *Ann Oncol* 1999; **10**: 317–21.

32. Montalban C, Castrillo JM, Lopez-Abente G et al, Other cancers in patients with gastric MALT lymphoma. *Leuk Lymphoma* 1999; **33**: 161–8.

33. Lamarque D, Gilbert T, Roudot-Thoraval F et al, Seroprevalence of eight *Helicobacter pylori* antigens among 182 patients with peptic ulcer, MALT gastric lymphoma or non-ulcer dyspepsia. Higher rate of seroreactivity against CagA and 35-kDa antigens in patients with peptic ulcer originating from Europe and Africa. *Eur J Gastroenterol Hepatol* 1999; **11**: 721–6.

34. Holly EA, Lele C, Bracci PM, McGrath MS, Case–control study of non-Hodgkin's lymphoma among women and heterosexual men in the San Francisco Bay Area, California. *Am J Epidemiol* 1999; **150**: 375–89.

35. Zhang S, Hunter DJ, Rosner BA et al, Dietary fat and protein in relation to risk of non-Hodgkin's lymphoma among women. *J Natl Cancer Inst* 1999; **91**: 1751–8.

36. Adami J, Gridley G, Nyren O et al, Sunlight and non-Hodgkin's lymphoma: a population-based cohort study in Sweden. *Int J Cancer* 1999; **80**: 641–5.

37. Hardell L, Eriksson M, A case–control study of non-Hodgkin lymphoma and exposure to pesticides. *Cancer* 1999; **85**: 1353–60.

38. Ruiz-Arguelles GJ, Velazquez BM, Apreza-Molina MG et al, Chronic lympho-cytic leukemia is infrequent in Mexican mestizos. *Int J Hematol* 1999; **69**: 253–5.

39. Mauro FR, Foa R, Giannarelli D et al, Clinical characteristics and outcome of young chronic lymphocytic leukemia patients: a single institution study of 204 cases. *Blood* 1999; **94**: 448–54.

40. Floderus B, Stenlund C, Persson T, Occupational magnetic field exposure and site specific cancer incidence: a Swedish cohort study. *Cancer Causes Control* 1999; **10**: 323–32.

41. Miligi L, Seniori CA, Crosignani P et al, Occupational, environmental, and life-style factors associated with the risk of hematolymphopoietic malignancies in women. *Am J Ind Med* 1999; **36**: 60–9.

42. Little MP, Weiss HA, Boice JDJ et al, Risks of leukemia in Japanese atomic bomb survivors, in women treated for cervical cancer, and in patients treated for ankylosing spondylitis. *Radiat Res* 1999; **152**: 280–92.

43. Ohyashiki JH, Abe K, Ojima T et al, Quantification of human herpesvirus 6 in healthy volunteers and patients with lymphoproliferative disorders by PCR–ELISA. *Leuk Res* 1999; **23**: 625–30.

44. Hamblin T, Davis Z, Gardiner S et al, Unmutated Ig V(H) genes are associated with a more aggressive form of chronic lymphocytic leukemia. *Blood* 1999; **94**: 1848–54.

45. Damle RN, Wasil T, Fais F et al, Ig V gene mutation status and CD38 expression as novel prognostic indicators in chronic lymphocytic leukemia. *Blood* 1999; **94**: 1840–7.

46. Levy U, Ugo V, Delmer A et al, Cyclin D1 overexpression allows identification of an aggressive subset of leukemic lymphoproliferative disorder. *Leukemia* 1999; **13**: 1343–51.

47. Callea V, Morabito F, Oliva BM et al, Surface CD14 positivity in B-cell chronic lymphocytic leukaemia is related to clinical outcome. *Br J Haematol* 1999; **107**: 347–52.

48. Molica S, Levato D, Cascavilla N et al, Clinico-prognostic implications of simultaneous increased serum levels of soluble CD23 and beta-2-microglobulin in B-cell chronic lymphocytic leukemia. *Eur J Haematol* 1999; **62**: 117–22.

49. Bevan S, Catovsky D, Marossy A et al, Linkage analysis for ATM in familial B cell chronic lymphocytic leukemia. *Leukemia* 1999; **13**: 1497–500.

50. Stankovic T, Weber P, Stewart G et al, Inactivation of ataxia telangiectasia mutated gene in B-cell chronic lymphocytic leukaemia. *Lancet* 1999; **353**: 26–9.

51. Sembries S, Pahl H, Stilgenbauer S et al, Reduced expression of adhesion molecules and cell signaling receptors by chronic lymphocytic leukemia cells with 11q deletion. *Blood* 1999; **93**: 624–31.

FURTHER READING

Multiple myeloma

Berenson JR, Vescio RA, HHV-8 is present in multiple myeloma patients. *Blood* 1999; **93**: 3157–66.

Bergsagel DE, Wong O, Bergsagel PL et al, Benzene and multiple myeloma: appraisal of the scientific evidence. *Blood* 1999; **94**: 1174–82.

Brown LM, Linet MS, Greenberg RS et al, Multiple myeloma and family history of cancer among blacks and whites in the U.S. *Cancer* 1999; **85**: 2385–90.

Cartwright RA, Gilman EA, Nicholson P, Allon D, Epidemiology of multiple myeloma in parts of England, 1984–1993. *Hematol Oncol* 1999; **17**: 31–8.

Tarte K, Chang Y, Klein B, Kaposi's sarcoma-associated herpesvirus and multiple myeloma: lack of criteria for causality. *Blood* 1999; **93**: 3159–63.

Hodgkin's disease

Flavell K, Constandinou C, Lowe D et al, Effect of material deprivation on Epstein–Barr virus infection in Hodgkin's disease in the west Midlands. *Br J Cancer* 1999; **80**: 604–8.

Jarrett RF, MacKenzie J, Epstein–Barr virus and other candidate viruses in the pathogenesis of Hodgkin's disease. *Semin Hematol* 1999; **36**: 260–9.

Khuder SA, Mutgi AB, Schaub EA, Tano BDK, Meta-analysis of Hodgkin's disease among farmers. *Scand J Work Environ Health* 1999; **225**: 436–41.

Nichols KE, Levitz S, Shannon KE et al, Heterozygous germline ATM mutations do not contribute to radiation-associated malignancies after Hodgkin's disease. *J Clin Oncol* 1999; **17**: 1259–66.

Rowlings PA, Curtis RE, Passweg JR et al, Increased incidence of Hodgkin's disease after allogeneic bone marrow transplantation. *J Clin Oncol* 1999; **17**: 3122–7.

2
The *BCL6* story

Finbarr E Cotter, Francesco Bertoni

INTRODUCTION

The observation that promiscuous translocations involving the chromosome 3q27 were frequently found in diffuse large B-cell lymphomas (DLBCL) and in follicular lymphomas (FL)[1–8] led to discovery of the *BCL6* gene (*B-cell lymphomas gene 6*, also known as *lymphoma-associated zinc finger 3, LAZ3*). Since then, much research has taken place to try and unravel the role of this gene. It is known that *BCL6* encodes for a 706-amino-acid 95 kDa nuclear phosphoprotein containing six C-terminal zinc-finger motifs, which act as DNA-binding domain, and an N-terminal bric-à-brac tramtrack broad complex/poxviruses and zinc fingers (BTP/POZ) domain, which is important for self and non-self protein–protein interactions, and for targeting of the protein to the nuclear dots.[1–5,7,9] At low levels, *BCL6* transcript can be found in skeletal muscles and lung tissues, but it is only specifically expressed at high levels in germinal centre B cells.[1–3,7,10] Both translocations and mutations involving the *BCL6* gene have been described.

BCL6 TRANSLOCATIONS ARE PROMISCUOUS

The *BCL6* locus is rearranged in 30–40% of DLBCL and in 10–20% of FL.[3,11–17] The breakpoints on chromosome 3q27 cluster within two regions: the 5′ flanking region spanning the promoter and the first non-coding exon or the first intron (major translocation cluster, MTC). The result is the juxtaposition of the *BCL6* full-length coding region (exons 2–10) to heterologous promoters derived from the other partner chromosomes. While the *BCL1, BCL2,* and c-*MYC* genes are always juxtaposed to immunoglobulin (Ig) heavy-chain (IgH) genes on 14q32 or light-chain (IgL) genes κ on 2p12 or λ on 22q11,[18] translocations involving *BCL6* affect heterologous loci.[12] The most common translocation remains the t(3;14)(q27;q32), juxtaposing the *BCL6* coding region to the IgH chain gene promoter.[19] Numerous additional partner genes have been identified; however, the *BCL6* coding region remains intact. The result of the t(3;4)(q27;p13) translocation is to fuse the *BCL6* gene to the *RhoH/TTF* gene, encoding a Rho GTPase enzyme involved in cytoskeleton organization.[20,21] Similarly, *BOB1/OBF1*, a B-cell-specific coactivator of octamer-binding transcription factors, is the partner gene in the t(3;11)(q27;q23).[22] The t(3;6)(q27;p21) translocation results in the *BCL6* coding region being juxtaposed to the *H4* histone gene.[23] The t(3;13)(q27;q14) revealed a *BCL6* fusion to the promoter of the *LCP1* gene encoding L-plastin, an actin-binding protein.[20] Xu and colleagues[24] cloned the *BCL6* fusion transcripts in five cases of primary gastric DLBCL. IgH were involved in three lymphomas, and IgLλ and the heat-shock protein 89 α gene (*HSP89A*) in the other two cases. A further 55 3q27 translocations were cloned by Akasaka and Coll.[25] Thirty cases involved Ig genes (IgH in 22, and IgL λ and κ genes in seven and one, respectively). Twenty-three involved non-Ig genes, such as *H4, HSP89A*, the heat-shock protein 90β gene (*HSP90B*), and *PIM-1* on 6p21.2, a serine/threonine protein kinase expressed primarily in cells of the haematopoietic and germ line cells. Finally, in another series of 14 cases,[26] IgH genes were the fusion partners in nine cases, while other partner genes were *PIM-1*, the MHC class II transactivator gene (*CIITA*), the eukaryotic initiation factor 4AII gene (*EIF4AII*), the transferring receptor gene (*TFRR*), and the *ikaros* genes. In general, all the partner genes involved in 3q27 translocations have expression patterns that differ from the germinal centre pattern normally found for *BCL6*, and probably determine abnormal persistence of *BCL6* expression beyond the germinal centre.

As with all chromosome abnormalities, it is of interest to determine whether or not the translocation is the primary event. Evidence suggests that the chromosome 3q27 abnormalities occur as primary cytogenetic events, even in cases expressing both a t(14;18)(q32;q21) and 3q27 translocations.[8,15,27–29] From the prognostic point of view, *BCL6* rearrangements do not seem to act as a poor prognostic factor in DLBCL.[11,27,30 32]

BCL6 MUTATIONS

In 1995, the *BCL6* 5′ non-coding region was shown to be the target of multiple, often biallelic, mutations in both FL and DLBCL cases, whether or not a translocation was present.[33] Subsequently, the same pattern of mutations was also detected in normal germinal centre B cells,[34,35] leading to much confusion regarding the role of these mutations in the pathogenesis of lymphoma. The *BCL6* mutations were at a high frequency similar to that occurring normally for somatic mutations within the immunoglobulin gene and at least tenfold greater than mutations detected for other genes such as c-*MYC*, the ribosomal small-subunit protein 14, β-globin or α-fetoprotein.[35] Peng et al[36] reported the *BCL6* analysis in 59 FL, 45 MALT lymphomas and 21 mantle cell lymphomas, detecting mutations in 42%, 42%, and 4.8% of the cases, respectively. Moreover, analogous mutations were found in 54% of normal germinal centre B cells and in 4% of normal mantle cells.

The presence of *BCL6* mutations in the different lymphoma subtypes is clearly shown in a large series of 308 B-cell neoplasms classified according to the Revised European–American Classification of Lymphoid Neoplasms (REAL)[37] and analysed by Capello and colleagues.[16] Mutations were absent or rare in tumours derived from precursor and antigen-virgin B cells (none in acute lymphoblastic leukaemias, 10% in mantle cell lymphomas). However, neoplasms of germinal centre or post germinal centre B cells demonstrated a pattern of mutation frequently seen in lymphoplasmacytoid lymphomas (40%), MALT lymphomas (33%), FL (60%), DLBCL (49%), and Burkitt's lymphomas (37%). Systemic nodal DLBCL, primary extranodal DLBCL, CD5+ DLBCL, CD30+ DLBCL, and primary splenic DLBCL all had the same frequency of *BCL6* mutations. This could suggest a similar histogenesis for these neoplasms.[16] In another paper from the same group,[38] both HIV-negative and HIV-positive cases of human herpesvirus 8/Kaposi's sarcoma-associated herpesvirus (HHV8/KSHV)-positive primary effusion lymphoma, another DLBCL subtype, showed *BCL6* mutations in 61% of the cases. Conversely, primary mediastinal DLCL with sclerosis had a low frequency of mutations (10%) – a clue to a different histogenetic pathway for this entity.[16] The detection of *BCL6* mutations in B-cell chronic lymphocytic leukaemias (CLL) (30%), small lymphocytic lymphomas (22%), and hairy cell leukaemias (25%)[16] supported the hypothesis that a fraction of these tumours might be related to germinal centre B cells. Mutations in *BCL6* share many characteristics with those found in Ig genes. They are not randomly distributed, occur at a very high frequency, are mostly single substitutions (transitions, in the first place), and are often clustered in short sequences. All of these data[34–36] indicate that the same hypermutation process active in Ig affinity maturation might also target *BCL6*. However, recent data showing that *BCL6* mutations are not actually associated with the presence of IgH chain gene somatic mutations in B-CLL goes against this hypothesis.[39] Moreover, if the *BCL6* mutation patterns are similar in both normal and neoplastic B cells derived from the germinal centre, then the vast majority of *BCL6* mutations detected in lymphomas could be irrelevant to the neoplastic process. Pasqualucci et al[40] have recently shown that some mutated *BCL6* alleles might have altered transcriptional activity. The *BCL6* 5′ noncoding region from six DLCBL and five Burkitt's lymphomas (corresponding to 20 mutated alleles) and from normal germinal centre B cells were linked to a reporter gene, and their transcriptional activity was evaluated in a transient transfection assay in two B-cell lymphoma lines. When compared with the wild-type allele, significant overexpression of the reporter gene was observed in 33% of the DLBCL-derived mutant alleles in both of transfected cell lines used. Three out of 6 DLBCL cases carried at least one overexpressed allele. Conversely, none of the constructs derived from Burkitt's lymphoma cases or normal germinal centre B cells gave abnormal transcriptional activity. In one case analysed in detail, the overexpression is due to a single nucleotide substitution within exon 1, affecting a *BCL6* DNA-binding site and preventing *BCL6* binding to its promoter region in vitro, suggesting that it may abrogate a *BCL6* negative autoregulatory circuit in vivo. Besides point mutations, the loss of regulatory sequences might even derive from internal deletions affecting intron 1, as reported in four cases.[41] Overall, these findings suggest that in certain cases, mutations within the BCL6 gene could play a role in the pathogenesis of lymphoma.

BCL6 EXPRESSION

Immunohistochemical data (reviewed by Falini et al[42]) show that germinal centre B cells, both centroblasts and centrocytes, show a strong nuclear positivity for BCL6 protein, with a diffuse or microgranular pattern. Conversely, mantle zone B cells, perisinusoidal and marginal zone B cells, plasma cells and precursor B cells all appear negative for BCL6 protein. A small subset of CD4$^+$ T cells and activated CD30$^+$ lymphoid cells may express BCL6. Analogously to their supposed normal counterparts and regardless of their 3q27 locus, FL, DBCL, Burkitt's lymphomas, and nodular lymphocyte-predominant Hodgkin's disease cells are strongly BCL6-positive. In the latter, the neoplastic cells are surrounded by BCL6$^+$/CD4$^+$ T cells. Mantle cell lymphomas, marginal zone B-cell lymphomas, and small lymphocytic/chronic lymphocytic leukaemias are negative for BCL6 immunostaining.[17,42] Raible and colleagues[43] reported BCL6 immunostaining data in a series of 72 lymphomas. All 31 FL were positive for BCL6, in contrast to only 1 out of 13 small lymphocytic lymphomas and 1 of 12 mantle cell lymphomas. Sixteen marginal zone B-cell lymphomas were all BCL6-negative. BCL6 immunostaining could be useful in differentiating FL from other small cell lymphomas. To underline the failure of monoclonal antibodies against BCL6 to discriminate between normal and translocated BCL6 forms, a recent paper[15] reported positive BCL6 immunostaining in 8 out of 13 (62%) DLBCL bearing the 3q27 translocation and in 33 of 39 (85%) without it.

THE ROLE OF BCL6

The role of BCL6 in germinal centre formation[44,45] has been suggested by experiments in the mouse, knocking out the gene. Despite normal B- and T-cell and lymphoid organ development, BCL6-deficient mice had a defect in T-cell-dependent antibody responses, due to a complete inability of the B cells to form germinal centres.[44,45] This is the site where immunoglobulin switch and affinity maturation should normally take place. Deficient mice also develop a multiorgan inflammatory response, characterized by infiltration of eosinophils and IgE-positive B cells.[44,45]

The positive role of BCL6 protein in germinal centre formation, and its possible role in oncogenesis in lymphomas, remain largely obscure. In addition, the proteins normally interacting and regulating BCL6 expression are still unknown. BCL6 appears as a strong transcriptional repressor, and it has been suggested that it plays a role in the regulation of apoptosis[46,47] through the CD40 molecule. In vitro activation of the B-cell receptor (BCR) by anti-IgM treatment, mimicking antigenic stimulation in absence of other co-factors, leads to apoptosis in EBV-negative Burkitt's lymphoma cell lines, representing the transformed counterparts of germinal centre B cells.[48] Apoptotic death is preceded by a rapid downregulation of BCL6 protein expression via its MAPK-mediated phosphorylation of specific serine residues followed by degradation by the ubiquitin–proteasome pathway.[48–50] Niu and colleagues[47] infected the RAMOS B-cell lymphoma line with a retroviral vector expressing mutant BCL6 proteins resistant to BCR-induced degradation due to mutations of MAPK phosphorylation sites or deletion of PEST motifs recognized by the ubiquitin–proteasome pathway. RAMOS cells expressing the mutant BCL6 proteins became resistant to BCR-induced death, and the degree of resistance correlated with the levels of constitutive BCL6 expression.[47] In the same in vitro model, signalling by CD40 or by its functional homolog EBV–LMP1 also led to BCL6 downregulation at transcriptional level.[7] Indeed, co-stimulation of B cells with CD40 and interleukin-4 (IL-4) downregulated BCL6 and up-regulated interferon-regulatory factor 4 (IRF4).[51] IRF4 is a transcription factor specific for lymphocytic lineage, and is known to be involved in the transactivation of both IgLκ and IgLλ chain enhancers and of CD20 and CD23b promoters.[52] IL-4 acts by binding to a membrane receptor, activating, via Janus kinases (JAKs), cytoplasmic signal transducers and activator of transcription (Stat) 6.[53] Tyrosine-phosphorylated Stat6 homodimerizes, and translocates to the nucleus, where it modulates transcription by binding distinct DNA sequences. BCL6, via the six C-terminal zinc-finger motifs, can bind to several DNA elements recognized by Stat6 and IRF4.[54] It can repress the IL-4-dependent induction of Ig germ-line ε transcripts. In fact, *BCL6*-deficient mice display an increased ability to class-switch to IgE in response to IL-4 in vitro, and exhibit a multi-organ inflammatory disease characterized by the presence of a large number of IgE+ B cells. The apparent dysregulation of IgE production is abolished in *BCL6*$^{-/-}$ *Stat6*$^{-/-}$ mice, further demonstrating that BCL6 regulation of Ig class switching is dependent upon Stat6 signalling. Germinal centre T cells express both CD40 ligand (CD154) and IL-4; thus they might provide successfully selected B cells with the necessary stimuli for their terminal stage differentiation.

Via its N-terminal BTP/POZ domain, BCL6 can interact with a complex comprising SMRT (silencing mediator of retinoid and thyroid receptor), mSIN3A and the histone deacetylase HDAC1.[54–58] The SMRT protein is a co-repressor recruited to DNA by BTP/POZ-domain/zinc-finger proteins, by nuclear receptors, such as the retinoid α receptor and the thyroid hormone receptor, and by the Mad/Max heterodimeric complexes. The whole co-repressor complex mediates DNA silencing by multiple mechanisms, which may include covalent modification of the chromatin template by the HDAC1 component and inhibitory interactions with transcription factors, mediated in part by the SMRT unit.

In lymphomas, BCL6 ectopic expression beyond the germinal centre might maintain a hypoacetylated chromatin structure for some genes, whose expression would be necessary for late B-cell differentiation. Moreover, BCL6 binds to proteins involved in other cell pathways. HDAC1 is recruited by Mad1 and pRb to repress the transcription of genes involved in cell cycle progression.[59] Thus, deregulation of BCL6 might disturb both cell differentiation and the cell cycle, sequestering the molecules common to other pathways. While the role of the BCL6 gene in the pathogenesis of lymphoma remains unclear, its role in both apoptosis and cell cycle pathways is being established. Future work will continue to establish the interaction with genes influencing the expression of BCL6 and the influence of BCL6 on downstream events in the germinal centre and the malignant cell. This in turn may permit us to understand the events predisposing this gene to translocation and mutation in both normal and abnormal B cells.

REFERENCES

1. Ye BH, Rao PH, Chaganti RS, Dalla-Favera R, Cloning of bcl-6, the locus involved in chromosome translocations affecting band 3q27 in B-cell lymphoma. Cancer Res 1993; 53: 2732–5.

2. Kerckaert JP, Deweindt C, Tilly H et al, LAZ3, a novel zinc-finger encoding gene, is disrupted by recurring chromosome 3q27 translocations in human lymphomas. Nature Genet 1993; 5: 66–70.

3. Ye BH, Lista F, Lo Coco F et al, Alterations of a zinc finger-encoding gene, BCL-6, in diffuse large-cell lymphoma. Science 1993; 262: 747–50.

4. Miki T, Kawamata N, Hirosawa S, Aoki N, Gene involved in the 3q27 translocation associated with B-cell lymphoma, BCL5, encodes a Kruppel-like zinc-finger protein. Blood 1994; 83: 26–32.

5. Baron BW, Nucifora G, McCabe N et al, Identification of the gene associated with the recurring chromosomal translocations t(3;14)(q27;q32) and t(3;22) (q27;q11) in B-cell lymphomas. Proc Natl Acad Sci USA 1993; 90: 5262–6.

6. Mitelman F, Mertens F, Johansson B, A breakpoint map of recurrent chromosomal rearrangements in human neoplasia. Nature Genet 1997; 15: 417–74.

7. Dalla-Favera R, Migliazza A, Chang CC et al, Molecular pathogenesis of B cell malignancy: the role of BCL-6. Curr Top Microbiol Immunol 1999; 246: 257–63.

8. Muramatsu M, Akasaka T, Kadowaki N et al, Rearrangement of the BCL6 gene in B-cell lymphoid neoplasms. Leukemia 1997; 11(Suppl 3): 318–20.

9. Dhordain P, Albagli O, Ansieau S et al, The BTB/POZ domain targets the LAZ3/BCL6 oncoprotein to nuclear dots and mediates homomerisation in vivo. Oncogene 1995; 11: 2689–97.

10. Cattoretti G, Chang CC, Cechova K et al, BCL-6 protein is expressed in germinal-center B cells. Blood 1995; 86: 45–53.

11. Vitolo U, Gaidano G, Botto B et al, Rearrangements of bcl-6, bcl-2, c-myc and 6q deletion in B-diffuse large-cell lymphoma: clinical relevance in 71 patients. Ann Oncol 1998; 9: 55–61.

12. Chen W, Iida S, Louie DC et al, Heterologous promoters fused to BCL6 by chromosomal translocations affecting band 3q27 cause its deregulated expression during B-cell differentiation. Blood 1998; 91: 603–7.

13. Otsuki T, Yano T, Clark HM et al, Analysis of LAZ3 (BCL-6) status in B-cell

non-Hodgkin's lymphomas: results of rearrangement and gene expression studies and a mutational analysis of coding sequences. *Blood* 1995; **85**: 2877–84.

14. Offit K, Lo Coco F, Louie DC et al. Rearrangement of the bcl-6 gene as a prognostic marker in diffuse large-cell lymphoma. *N Engl J Med* 1994; **331**: 74–80.

15. Skinnider BF, Horsman DE, Dupuis B, Gascoyne RD, Bcl-6 and Bcl-2 protein expression in diffuse large B-cell lymphoma and follicular lymphoma: correlatation with 3q27 and 18q21 chromosomal abnormalities. *Hum Pathol* 1999; **30**: 803–8.

16. Capello D, Vitolo U, Pasqualucci L et al, Distribution and pattern of BCL-6 mutations throughout the spectrum of B-cell neoplasia. *Blood* 2000; **95**: 651–9.

17. Gaidano G, Capello D, Gloghini A et al, Frequent mutation of bcl-6 proto-oncogene in high grade, but not low grade, MALT lymphomas of the gastrointestinal tract. *Haematologica* 1999; **84**: 582–8.

18. Cotter FE, Molecular pathology of lymphomas. *Cancer Surv* 1993; **16**: 157–74.

19. Ye BH, Chaganti S, Chang CC et al, Chromosomal translocations cause deregulated BCL6 expression by promoter substitution in B cell lymphoma. *EMBO J* 1995; **14**: 6209–17.

20. Galiegue-Zouitina S, Quief S, Hildebrand MP et al, Nonrandom fusion of L-plastin (LCP1) and LAZ3 (BCL6) genes by t(3;13)(q27;q14) chromosome translocation in two cases of B-cell non-Hodgkin lymphoma. *Genes Chromosomes Cancer* 1999; **26**: 97–105.

21. Dallery E, Galiegue-Zouitina S, Collyn-d'Hooghe M et al, TTF, a gene encoding a novel small G protein, fuses to the lymphoma-associated LAZ3 gene by t(3;4) chromosomal translocation. *Oncogene* 1995; **10**: 2171–8.

22. Galiegue-Zouitina S, Quief S, Hildebrand MP et al, The B cell transcriptional coactivator BOB1/OBF1 gene fuses to the LAZ3/BCL6 gene by t(3;11)(q27;q23.1)

chromosomal translocation in a B cell leukemia line (Karpas 231). *Leukemia* 1996; **10**: 579–87.

23. Akasaka T, Miura I, Takahashi N, Akasaka H et al, A recurring translocation, t(3;6)(q27;p21), in non-Hodgkin's lymphoma results in replacement of the 5′ regulatory region of BCL6 with a novel H4-histone gene. *Cancer Res* 1997; **57**: 7–12.

24. Xu WS, Liang RH, Srivastava G, Identification and characterization of BCL6 translocation partner genes in primary gastric high-grade B-cell lymphoma: heat shock protein 89 alpha is a novel fusion partner gene of BCL6. *Genes Chromosomes Cancer* 2000; **27**: 69–75.

25. Akasaka H, Akasaka T, Ohno H, Uchiyama T, Diverse molecular anatomy of BCL6 translocations leading to deregulated expression of the gene. *Blood* 1999; **94** (10 Suppl 1): 273.

26. Yoshida S, Kaneita Y, Aoki Y et al, Identification of heterologous translocation partner genes fused to the BCL6 gene in diffuse large B-cell lymphomas: 5′-RACE and LA-PCR analyses of biopsy samples. *Oncogene* 1999; **18**: 7994–9.

27. Kramer MH, Hermans J, Wijburg E et al, Clinical relevance of BCL2, BCL6, and MYC rearrangements in diffuse large B-cell lymphoma. *Blood* 1998; **92**: 3152–62.

28. Daudignon A, Bisiau H, Le Baron F et al, Four cases of follicular lymphoma with t(14;18)(q23;q21) and t(3;4)(q27;p13) with LAZ3 (BCL6) rearrangement. *Cancer Genet Cytogenet* 1999; **111**: 157–60.

29. Au WY, Gascoyne RD, Viswanatha DS et al, Concurrent chromosomal alterations at 3q27, 8q24 and 18q21 in B-cell lymphomas. *Br J Haematol* 1999; **105**: 437–40.

30. Bastard C, Deweindt C, Kerckaert JP et al, LAZ3 rearrangements in non-Hodgkin's lymphoma: correlation with histology, immunophenotype, karyotype, and clinical outcome in 217 patients. *Blood* 1994; **83**: 2423–7.

31. Liang R, Chan WP, Kwong YL et al, High incidence of BCL-6 gene rearrange-

ment in diffuse large B-cell lymphoma of primary gastric origin. *Cancer Genet Cytogenet* 1997; **97**: 114–18.

32. Offit K, Louis DC, Parsa NZ et al, BCL6 gene rearrangement and other cytogenetic abnormalities in diffuse large cell lymphoma. *Leuk Lymphoma* 1995; **20**: 85–9.

33. Migliazza A, Martinotti S, Chen W et al, Frequent somatic hypermutation of the 5′ noncoding region of the BCL6 gene in B-cell lymphoma. *Proc Natl Acad Sci USA* 1995; **92**: 12520–4.

34. Pasqualucci L, Migliazza A, Fracchiolla N et al, BCL-6 mutations in normal germinal center B cells: evidence of somatic hypermutation acting outside Ig loci. *Proc Natl Acad Sci USA* 1998; **95**: 11816–21.

35. Shen HM, Peters A, Baron B et al, Mutation of BCL-6 gene in normal B cells by the process of somatic hypermutation of Ig genes. *Science* 1998; **280**: 1750–2.

36. Peng HZ, Du MQ, Koulis A et al, Nonimmunoglobulin gene hypermutation in germinal center B cells. *Blood* 1999; **93**: 2167–72.

37. Harris NL, Jaffe ES, Stein H et al, A revised European–American classification of lymphoid neoplasms: a proposal from the International Lymphoma Study Group. *Blood* 1994; **84**: 1361–92.

38. Gaidano G, Capello D, Cilia AM et al, Genetic characterization of HHV-8/KSHV-positive primary effusion lymphoma reveals frequent mutations of BCL6: implications for disease pathogenesis and histogenesis. *Genes Chromosomes Cancer* 1999; **24**: 16–23.

39. Sahota SS, Davis Z, Hamblin TJ, Stevenson FK, Somatic mutation of bcl-6 genes can occur in the absence of V(H) mutations in chronic lymphocytic leukemia. *Blood* 2000; **95**: 3534–40.

40. Pasqualucci L, Migliazza A, Ye BH et al, Transcriptional deregulation of mutated BCL-6 alleles in diffuse large cell lymphomas. *Blood* 1999; **94** (10 Suppl 1): 58.

41. Nakamura Y, Saito K, Furusawa S, Analysis of internal deletions within the BCL6 gene in B-cell non-Hodgkin's lymphoma. *Br J Haematol* 1999; **105**: 274–7.

42. Falini B, Fizzotti M, Pileri S et al, Bcl-6 protein expression in normal and neoplastic lymphoid tissues. *Ann Oncol* 1997; **8**: 101–4.

43. Raible MD, Hsi ED, Alkan S, Bcl-6 protein expression by follicle center lymphomas. A marker for differentiating follicle center lymphomas from the other low-grade lymphoproliferative disorders. *Am J Clin Pathol* 1999; **112**: 101–7.

44. Ye BH, Cattoretti G, Shen Q et al, The BCL-6 proto-oncogene controls germinal-centre formation and Th2-type inflammation, *Nature Genet* 1997; **16**: 161–70.

45. Dent AL, Shaffer AL, Yu X et al, Control of inflammation, cytokine expression, and germinal center formation by BCL-6. *Science* 1997; **276**: 589–92.

46. Staudt LM, Dent AL, Shaffer AL, Yu X, Regulation of lymphocyte cell fate decisions and lymphomagenesis by BCL-6. *Int Rev Immunol* 1999; **18**: 381–403.

47. Niu H, Pietrafesa R, Cattoretti G, Dalla Favera R, The BCL-6 proto-oncogene controls apoptosis in B cells. *Blood* 1999; **94** (10 Suppl 1): 693.

48. Niu H, Ye BH, Dalla-Favera R, Antigen receptor signaling induces MAP kinase-mediated phosphorylation and degradation of the BCL-6 transcription factor. *Genes Dev* 1998; **12**: 1953–61.

49. Moriyama M, Yamochi T, Semba K et al, BCL-6 is phosphorylated at multiple sites in its serine- and proline-clustered region by mitogen-activated protein kinase (MAPK) in vivo. *Oncogene* 1997; **14**: 2465–74.

50. Allman D, Jain A, Dent A et al, BCL-6 expression during B-cell activation. *Blood* 1996; **87**: 5257–68.

51. Gupta S, Jiang M, Anthony A, Pernis AB, Lineage-specific modulation of interleukin 4 signaling by interferon regulatory factor 4. *J Exp Med* 1999; **190**: 1837–48.

52. Mamane Y, Heylbroeck C, Genin P et al, Interferon regulatory factors: the next generation. *Gene* 1999; **237**: 1–14.

53. Nelms K, Huang H, Ryan J et al, Interleukin-4 receptor signalling mechanisms and their biological significance. *Adv Exp Med Biol* 1998; **452**: 37–43.

54. Harris MB, Chang CC, Berton MT et al, Transcriptional repression of Stat6-dependent interleukin-4-induced genes by BCL-6: specific regulation of iepsilon transcription and immunoglobulin E switching. *Mol Cell Biol* 1999; **19**: 7264–75.

55. Deweindt C, Albagli O, Bernardin F et al, The LAZ3/BCL6 oncogene encodes a sequence-specific transcriptional inhibitor: a novel function for the BTB/POZ domain as an autonomous repressing domain. *Cell Growth Differ* 1995; **6**: 1495–503.

56. Dhordain P, Albagli O, Lin RJ et al, Corepressor SMRT binds the BTB/POZ repressing domain of the LAZ3/BCL6 oncoprotein. *Proc Natl Acad Sci USA* 1997; **94**: 10762–7.

57. Dhordain P, Lin RJ, Quief S et al, The LAZ3 (BCL-6) oncoprotein recruits a SMRT/mSIN3A/histone deacetylase containing complex to mediate transcriptional repression. *Nucleic Acids Res* 1998; **26**: 4645–51.

58. David G, Alland L, Hong SH et al, Histone deacetylase associated with mSin3A mediates repression by the acute promyelocytic leukemia-associated PLZF protein. *Oncogene* 1998; **16**: 2549–56.

59. Jacobson S, Pillus L, Modifying chromatin and concepts of cancer. *Curr Opin Genet Dev* 1999; **9**: 175–84.

3
Hodgkin's disease

Dennis L Cooper, Stuart Seropian

INTRODUCTION

The past several years have been marked by substantial evolution in the treatment of Hodgkin's disease (HD). Most noticeably, a greater proportion of patients with early-stage disease are now treated initially with chemotherapy, and radiation has assumed more of an adjuvant role. This shift in treatment has been driven by a greater awareness of the long-term complications of radiation and the availability of chemotherapy that does not cause infertility or leukemia. In patients with advanced disease, the use of ABVD and hybrid regimens appears to be giving way to more intensive chemotherapy. The current enthusiasm for more aggressive regimens reflects the unsatisfactory ceiling in cure rates that has been achieved with standard combination chemotherapy coincident with the markedly improved ability to support patients through more intensive therapy with the use of growth factors. For similar reasons, high-dose therapy supported with peripheral blood stem cells has moved from a treatment of last resort to the therapy of choice for patients who relapse after standard chemotherapy, regardless of the length of the original remission.

Unfortunately, changes in treatment have until now proceeded independently of advances in the biology of HD. One possible exception to the latter observation is in patients with lymphocyte-predominant HD (LPHD), where the finding of CD20 expression on the characteristic tumor cells may provide an attractive treatment option in a group of patients for whom standard treatment may have been worse than the disease. Nevertheless, as the desire to reduce long-term complications in patients with more favorable prognosis disease has become almost as important as devising new strategies to cure the 30–40% of patients not cured with standard therapy, it is hoped that molecular profiles of tumor cells will replace surrogate clinical features as a tool on which to base treatment.

In the present review, recent advances in the biology of HD will be presented particularly as they relate to pathogenesis and treatment. Subsequently, the 'standard' treatment of early- and advanced-stage Hodgkin's disease will be discussed, with special attention given to ongoing clinical trials and to papers published within the past year. The use of high-dose therapy will be primarily discussed in the context of disease that is resistant to or recurs after chemotherapy.

Finally, recent data on newer imaging strategies and opportunities for 'response-adapted treatment' are briefly highlighted.

UPDATE ON BIOLOGY OF HODGKIN'S DISEASE

Micromanipulation techniques that allow isolation of single Hodgkin's Reed–Sternberg (HRS) cells from tissue samples have provided convincing evidence that the HRS cell is of B-cell lineage. Building on this observation, two reports in 1999 suggested that HRS cells are, in fact, derived from germinal center B cells. Brauninger et al,[1] capitalizing on a rare clinical scenario, isolated single HRS cells and malignant B-cell lymphoma cells in two patients who had both HD and B-cell non-Hodgkin's lymphoma (NHL). In one patient, both malignancies were found at the same time, while in the second patient, HD was diagnosed several years after a prior diagnosis of T-cell-rich, B-cell NHL. Using seminested polymerase chain reaction (PCR), the investigators identified and sequenced the rearranged immunoglobulin heavy- and light-chain variable-region genes. The gene rearrangements from the HRS and NHL cells and the somatic mutations within those genes were compared. In both cases, the same clonal V-gene rearrangements were found, thereby indicating a common B-cell precursor. All rearrangements carried somatic mutations, some of which were shared by the HRS and NHL cells and some of which were restricted to only one or other of the tumors. Similar findings were reported by Marafioti et al[2] in a patient with advanced HD and subsequent follicular NHL that was diagnosed two years after remission of HD. The presence of identical immunoglobulin gene rearrangements and the finding of both shared and unique somatic mutations provide strong evidence that both tumors originated from a common germinal center B cell but that the subsequent unique transforming events determined the nature (HD versus B-cell lymphoma) of the resultant malignancy.

It has long been recognized that HRS cells exist in tissues with a unique histologic background characterized by a mixed inflammatory infiltrate with prominent eosinophils and sclerosis. These features, in association with B symptoms, have been theorized to be the result of abnormal cytokine secretion either by HRS cells or by other cells found in the tumor tissue. Kapp et al[3] used a microchip array with 950 cDNA segments from genes commonly expressed in either inflammatory or malignant states to characterize the cytokine profile of HRS cells. Patterns of gene expression in two HD cell lines were than compared with a control Epstein–Barr virus (EBV)-infected lymphoblastoid cell line. HD cells were found to express relatively high levels of a number of genes, most notably interleukin (IL)-13 and IL-5. Further studies on lymph node biopsy samples from four patients with nodular sclerosis HD, which included immunohistochemistry and in situ hybridization with an RNA probe for IL-13, confirmed localization to the HRS cells. Finally, the investigators demonstrated that a neutralizing antibody to IL-13 was capable of inhibiting proliferation of an HD cell line in a dose-dependent manner. Although these findings were the result of in vitro experiments from two cell lines, and should therefore be interpreted with some caution, a number of the identified biological properties of IL-13 are consistent with the pathologic observations of HD, including the presence of significant numbers of Th2-type lymphocytes in proximity to the HRS cells as well as the presence of fibrosis, which is thought to occur by stimulation of the fibroblast by IL-13. Whether IL-13 plays a primary role in the pathogenesis and/or clinical progression of HD remains to be demonstrated, although these findings suggest that it is a logical target for both new prognostic and experimental treatment strategies.

Using a novel approach, Cossman et al[4] attempted to define the regulated gene expression profile of single HRS cells, HD-derived cell lines, and HD tissues. In this interesting study, cDNA libraries were prepared from HRS cells and sequenced, yielding thousands of sequences for comparison with other cell types using worldwide data from GenBank. Of note, a number of B-cell-associated genes were found in high frequency in Hodgkin's cells, including immunoglobulin genes and the B-cell-associated antigen CD20. The frequency of expressed sequences in HRS were compared with a number of other cell types, including dendritic cells. In contrast to the similarities in gene expression with germinal B cells, there were substantial differences in the expressed sequences with dendritic cells. These data provide further evidence of the B-cell lineage of HRS cells. However, a number of genes not known to be expressed in HD or germinal center B cells were also overexpressed. For example, the melanoma tumor-associated antigen MAGE-4a was found in HRS cells with a relative frequency 219 times that of other cell types. As MAGE proteins may provide an excellent target for cytotoxic T lymphocytes, the observation of overexpression of MAGE-4a, if confirmed, might be used to develop immunologic programs to treat HD.

In a study that is perhaps of more immediate utility, Hasse et al[5] searched for evidence of clonal loss of heterozygosity (LOH) in HRS cells. In this analysis, DNA from microdissected HRS cells from seven patients was subjected to a microsatellite PCR assay to identify LOH at loci known from the cytogenetics literature to be deleted in a nonrandom fashion in HD patients. PCR was also performed to detect clonal immunoglobulin gene rearrangements in four of the patients. Six of the seven patients showed clonal LOH at one to three loci, and all four patients studied had clonal immunoglobulin gene rearrangements. Study of normal tissue (buccal mucosa or bystander lymphocytes) showed a constitutional microsatellite pattern indicating that LOH was specific to the HRS cells. This study again provides evidence for the clonality of HD, and suggests that tumor suppressor genes may play a role in the molecular pathogenesis of HD. Further characterization of these loci is eagerly awaited.

EARLY-STAGE DISEASE

A survey of ongoing clinical trials for early-stage Hodgkin's disease reflects the growing movement toward the use of combined-modality therapy (CMT, Table 3.1). Several factors have played a role in this treatment shift. First, the results of clinical trials and a recent meta-analysis have shown the superiority of CMT compared with radiation in curing patients with clinical stage I–II disease.[6] In fact, in the EORTC H6 trial, patients with unfavorable prognostic factors treated with CMT had a superior disease-free survival than a more favorable group of patients treated with radiation.[7] Secondly, it has not been possible to simultaneously reduce radiation fields and to avoid staging laparotomy without sustaining an unacceptable incidence of recurrence. For example, in the EORTC H7 trial, a group of 'very favorable', clinically staged patients (female gender, stage IA, lymphocyte-predominant or nodular sclerosis histology, no massive mediastinal disease), who constituted only 6% of all stage IA and IIA patients, were treated with mantle field radiation to a dose of 36–40 Gy. The disease-free survival rate was only 68% at six years, causing the EORTC to abandon mantle field radiation even in this very favorable group with CMT.[8] Similarly, Wirth et al[9] recently summarized their results in patients with clinical stage I–II disease who were given mantle field radiation in the years between 1969 and 1994. Even when the analysis was restricted to patients with a favorable clinical profile, the disease-free survival rate was only 70–73% overall, and in patients with stage II disease it was 48–57%. The authors concluded that more intensive therapy was required for patients with clinical stage II (CS II) disease, excepting those with lymphocyte-predominant histology.

Equally important to the development of the current level of enthusiasm for CMT with low-dose radiation therapy has been the recognition of late adverse effects (solid tumors and cardiovascular disease) after higher doses of radiation at a time when chemotherapy regimens are available that do not appear to cause infertility or leukemia. In fact, several studies suggest that in CMT programs, radiation doses can be lowered and treatment fields reduced to the involved field without an increase in relapse rates.[6,10–12] As CMT with low-dose radiation has not been implicated in the development of solid tumors or cardiovascular disease,[13–15] this treatment strategy may substantially reduce the incidence of late toxicity. Similarly, chemotherapy can be abbreviated in CMT programs, thereby reducing the potential for an adverse interaction with radiation as well as the cumulative toxicity from each drug and overall treatment time.[11,12] The use of chemotherapy obviates the need for surgical staging, which, in combination with the use of lower doses and smaller fields of radiation, should decrease the incidence of hyposplenism, an important cause of late sepsis.

The ongoing European studies should better define the extent to which chemotherapy can be shortened, as well as the minimum dose of adjuvant radiation that is required after abbreviated chemotherapy.

Table 3.1 Selected current trials for favorable, early-stage Hodgkin's disease

Study group	Trial[a]	Laparotomy	Comments[a]
EORTC H9	6 × EBVP + 36 Gy IF 6 × EBVP + 20 Gy IF 6 × EBVP	No	Tests whether radiation improves control. EBVP previously shown to be less active than MOPP/ABVD.
GHSG HD10	4 × ABVD + 30 Gy IF 4 × ABVD + 20 Gy IF 2 × ABVD + 30 Gy IF 2 × ABVD + 20 Gy IF	No	Optimal chemotherapy used. Study should give answer regarding duration of chemotherapy and dose of radiation therapy.
NCI-C/ECOG	STNI 4–6 × ABVD	Optional	Does not include combined-modality arm. Study size probably precludes showing difference in overall survival.
Stanford	Stanford V + 30 Gy IF	No	Eight weeks of chemotherapy. Data on male sterility, leukemia important.
POG	DBVE + 25.5 Gy IF ± dexrazoxane	Optional	Response-adapted treatment. Is there really a need for dexrazoxane? Risk of leukemia owing to etoposide.

[a] EBVP, epirubicin, bleomycin, vinblastine, prednisone; IF, involved field; ABVD, doxorubicin, bleomycin, vinblastine, dacarbazine; STNI, subtotal nodal irradiation; Stanford V, mechlorethamine, doxorubicin, vinblastine, vincristine, bleomycin, etoposide, prednisone (plus granulocyte colony-stimulating factor for dose reduction, delay); DBVE, doxorubicin, bleomycin, vincristine, etoposide; MOPP, mechlorethamine, vincristine, procarbazine, prednisone.

An important question that has surfaced in recent years is whether patients with LPHD should be treated like other patients with early-stage disease. Clinically, LPHD is more common in men than women, rarely involves the mediastinum, and is much less likely to be associated with stage III–IV disease than other histologies of HD. Characteristic lymphocyte and histiocyte cells (L&H or 'popcorn' cells) generally do not stain for Leu-M1 or Ki-1 antigens, but do stain positively for the B-cell marker CD20, thus distinguishing LPHD from

Table 3.2 Lymphocyte-predominant Hodgkin's disease is not similar to follicular small cell non-Hodgkin's lymphoma

Diagnosis	Age	Stage	Curability with standard treatment	Transformation to high-grade lymphoma?
Follicular small cell lymphoma	Generally older age groups	III–IV	Advanced-stage incurable	Yes
Lymphocyte-predominant Hodgkin's disease	Usually adolescent, young adults	I–II	70–80% disease-free survival	?

other types of HD, including the morphologically identical entity of lymphocyte-rich classic HD (LRCHD). Some investigators have suggested that LPHD is more similar to follicular small cell lymphoma than to classic HD because of the indolent clinical course and B-cell phenotype. On the other hand, there are very important differences (Table 3.2).

Traditionally, patients with LPHD have been treated like other patients with HD. However, because of the low incidence of disease-specific mortality and the results of one small study in which some patients did well without initial treatment,[16] some have questioned whether such patients should be treated less aggressively, if at all.

In an effort to further define the pathology, clinical presentation, response to therapy, and long-term follow-up of patients with LPHD, 426 patients with a diagnosis of LPHD from 17 centers in Europe and North America were analyzed.[17] After immunostaining studies, 51% retained the diagnosis of LPHD and 27% of cases were reclassified as LRCHD. The remaining cases were eliminated from further study because they showed classic HD, NHL, or reactive lesions, or had technically inadequate samples. Survival and failure-free survival were excellent and similar for LPHD and LRCHD, but were not significantly different for stage-comparable patients with classic HD. As a result, the better prognosis overall for patients with LPHD and LRCHD compared with classic HD is probably due to the tendency for the former groups to present with earlier-stage disease. The incidence of relapse was 21% in the LPHD group, compared with 17% in the LRCHD cohort. Interestingly, nearly one-quarter of the patients who relapsed in the LPHD group suffered subsequent relapses, compared with 5% of patients who relapsed with LRCHD. Despite the higher incidence of multiple relapses in the LPHD group, survival was excellent. Importantly, deaths from HD were less common than deaths attributed to treatment (second malignancies, cardiovascular disease) in patients with both LPHD and LRCHD.

The authors appropriately concluded that current treatment programs (usually including extended-field radiation) for patients with LPHD and LRCHD might not be optimal in terms of late toxicity. Nevertheless, as discussed above, the same conclusion can be drawn about treatment with wide-field radiation for other patients with early-stage HD, and it seems likely that newer CMT programs should cause far less long-term toxicity with at least comparable cure rates as extended-field radiation alone. Thus, the authors stated intention of performing a randomized trial in patients with stage I LPHD comparing immediate treatment versus a 'watch-and-wait' strategy is puzzling, since their own data suggest that both LPHD and LRCHD are curable diseases in approximately 70–80% of cases. Perhaps a more appropriate study would compare involved-field radiation with current CMT protocols. Because mediastinal involvement is uncommon in patients with LPDH and LRCHD, patients receiving involved-field radiation should not experience a heightened risk of cardiovascular complications and breast and lung cancer.

Another alternative treatment that will undoubtedly be tested in patients with LPHD will be the use of rituximab, a monoclonal antibody directed against the CD20 antigen. Rituximab should theoretically be effective in patients with LPHD because of the expression of CD20 in the L&H cells. In contrast, the malignant cells in LRCHD and classic HD do not express CD20, and rituximab would not be expected to be an effective treatment in these patient groups. The most appropriate patient population (newly diagnosed versus recurrent disease) to test the efficacy of rituximab remains to be determined.

ADVANCED DISEASE

The results of recent randomized trials show that ABVD (doxorubicin, bleomycin vinblastine, and dacarbazine) is superior to MOPP (mechlorethamine, vincristine, procarbazine, and prednisone), and at least as effective as MOPP alternating with ABVD or the use of the MOPP/ABV (doxorubicin, bleomycin, and vinblastine) hybrid.[18–20] Because of the potential for MOPP (or similar programs) to cause myelodysplasia and sterility, ABVD has become the standard regimen for patients with advanced disease in the USA. Nevertheless, approximately 40% of patients with stage III–IV disease will relapse or not respond to treatment, and the failure rate is considerably higher in some subsets of patients. As a result, there has been considerable interest in developing more effective regimens and in more precisely identifying patients with advanced disease who would be appropriate candidates for more intensive therapy at the time of diagnosis.

The increasing ability to support patients with hematopoietic growth factors and/or stem cells has facilitated the safe development of more intensive programs. For example, the German Hodgkin's Study Group showed that, in comparison with the standard regimen COPP (cyclophosphamide, vincristine, procarbazine, and prednisone)/ABVD, treatment with a dose-escalated version of BEACOPP (bleomycin, etoposide, doxorubicin, cyclophosphamide, vincristine, procarbazine, and prednisone) resulted in a superior freedom from progression and nearly eliminated the occurrence of disease progression during therapy.[21,22] Survival also appeared to be improved, but the difference is not yet statistically significant. An ongoing study will compare dose-escalated BEACOPP with standard-dose BEACOPP. Similarly, Carella et al[23] showed in a small study of 22 patients with 'poor-prognosis' Hodgkin's disease who entered remission after MOPP/ABVD that 17 patients remained in remission after a course of consolidative high-dose chemotherapy/autologous bone marrow rescue. A randomized trial that will test the benefit of early high-dose therapy/autologous stem cell rescue is currently in progress in Europe and an Intergroup trial is planned in the USA.

Despite the relative ease and safety with which patients can currently be treated with highly myelosuppressive chemotherapy, thus far there has not been a consensus on which patients with HD should be considered for more intensive therapy as part of initial treatment. This issue is particularly important because of the young age of most of the patients and the likelihood that such intensive therapy will result in a very high incidence of sterility/infertility and a measurable risk of myelodysplasia (MDS)/acute non-lymphocytic leukemia, complications that are rare after the use of conventional programs such as ABVD. As a result, there is substantial interest in creating a prognostic index similar to the one in use for NHL.

A study from the International Prognostic Factors Project for Advanced Hodgkin's disease identified seven adverse independent factors (albumin <4 g/dl, hemoglobin <10.5 g/dl male sex, age 45, stage IV disease, leukocytosis, and lymphocytopenia).[24] However, less than 20% of patients had five or more adverse factors, and only 7% had a prognostic index that predicted that the patient was more likely to relapse than to remain free from disease progression. Thus, one important conclusion of this scoring system is that it failed to identify a substantial number of patients who might benefit from more intensive treatment.

Two publications in 1999 described other potentially important prognostic factors. Sarris et al[25] found a significantly worse failure-free survival (60% versus 91%) in patients who had high levels of IL-10 expression versus those with low levels. IL-10 might promote treatment failure by inhibiting chemotherapy-induced apoptosis and by causing a subtle defect in T-cell-mediated immunity. Although the authors implied that IL-10 expression was potentially linked to EBV infection, this study did not correlate IL-10 level with molecular evidence of EBV infection. Moreover, a paper by Murray et al[26] suggests that EBV-associated HD is not associated with treatment resistance. They performed in situ hybridization assays for EBV-encoded early RNAs (EBERs) on tumor samples from 190 adult patients with advanced disease. The complete response rate and two-year failure-free survival of EBV-positive patients in this study were significantly better than those of EBV-negative patients. The latter results suggest that the negative impact of IL-10 on failure-free survival observed by Sarris et al[25] was probably not due to underlying EBV infection. With respect to the importance of these two studies on newly diagnosed patients, it is important to note that neither prognostic factor has been validated in a prospectively performed study. More importantly, these factors (IL-10 and EBV) did not strongly discriminate between patients who did well and those who did poorly with conventional therapy. Thus, the selection of patients for more intensive therapy at the time of diagnosis remains difficult and controversial.

RECURRENT DISEASE AFTER CHEMOTHERAPY

Independent of the length of initial remission, most patients who relapse after chemotherapy today are generally considered for salvage chemotherapy followed by high-dose therapy and stem cell rescue.[27] Several factors have lowered the enthusiasm for retreatment with conventional chemotherapy even in patients with initial long (over one year) remissions. First, high-dose therapy has become considerably safer and less expensive, with many patients now treated in the outpatient setting and with most experienced centers reporting a mortality rate less than 5%. Secondly, as most patients are now initially treated with ABVD or a combination of a MOPP-like regimen with ABVD, the choices for conventional treatment have been considerably reduced. Retreatment with anthracycline-based regimens is limited by the potential for cumulative heart toxicity, particularly if the patient has previously received mediastinal radiation. Similarly, while MOPP-like regimens may effect a response in patients who relapse after ABVD, their potential for causing MDS leukemia and inhibiting future stem cell collection have made this an unattractive option except in patients too ill to undergo other therapy. Finally, there are minimal long-term data that support the efficacy of conventional salvage therapy in patients treated with current programs. Thus, while some patients who relapsed after MOPP may have been cured with ABVD or by MOPP again, similar long-term data are not available for patients who have relapsed after ABVD or ABVD alternating with a MOPP-like regimen.

With respect to salvage chemotherapy prior to high-dose therapy/stem cell rescue, a recent paper from the MD Anderson Cancer Center suggests that the regimen ASHAP (doxorubicin, methylprednisolone, high-dose cytosine arabinoside, and cisplatin) was safe and highly effective (34% complete response rate and 36% partial response rate) in an unfavorable group of patients.[28] Patients with a partial or complete response after two cycles of therapy had a third cycle of treatment prior to high-dose therapy and stem cell rescue. Factors that predicted a poor response to ASHAP included B symptoms at relapse and a duration of response to the most recent previous therapy of less than six months. Interestingly, 60% of patients who achieved a negative gallium scan after ASHAP became long-term survivors after high-dose therapy/autologous stem cell rescue, compared with 35% in patients with persistent positive scans.

None of the 17 patients whose disease failed to respond to ASHAP became long-term survivors, suggesting that high-dose therapy may not be warranted in patients who fail treatment with this program. Although these results clearly identify ASHAP as an effective regimen, it is not clear that ASHAP is more effective than the similar regimen ESHAP (with etoposide instead of doxorubicin) which was also recently reported to achieve a 73% response rate,[29] or to other regimens such as ifosfamide/vinorelbine,[30] DHAP (dexamethasone, high-dose cytosine arabinoside, and cisplatin),[31] or EPOCH (etoposide, vincristine, doxorubicin, cyclophosphamide, and prednisone).[32]

One of the weaknesses of the high-dose therapy/autologous stem cell literature is the lack of comparative data on high-dose programs. At present, most patients are treated with either BEAM (carmustine, etoposide, cytosine arabinoside, and melphalan) or CBV (cyclophosphamide, carmustine, and etoposide). Although MDS and leukemia are feared potential complications of high-dose therapy, in fact most studies do not suggest that high-dose chemotherapy is a major risk factor in the development of MDS/leukemia. In a recent paper, Harrison et al[33] compared the incidence of MDS in HD patients who received a transplant and BEAM with the incidence in patients who received conventional therapy alone. Their analysis showed that the risk of MDS was directly related to the amount of therapy prior to BEAM but that the administration of BEAM did not confer a statistically significant independent risk. The Nebraska group had previously shown that MDS was restricted to patients who received total-body irradiation (TBI) as part of the preparative program[34] – a finding supported by the substantial risk of MDS in patients with follicular lymphoma transplanted in first remission after a preparative regimen that included TBI.[35] Taken together, these studies do not suggest that the fear of MDS should be used as a reason not to proceed to high-dose chemotherapy.

REFRACTORY DISEASE

In contrast to the situation in patients with NHL, where data show that refractory disease is not curable with high-dose therapy,[36] there is a growing literature, including several publications in 1999, suggesting that a significant number of patients with primary refractory HD can be cured with high-dose therapy. Using a large French database, Andre et al[37] analyzed 86 patients who underwent transplant either because they had progressive disease during first-line therapy (78 patients) or had less than a complete response and relapsed within three months of completing treatment (8 patients). These selection criteria thereby excluded patients who had residual radiographic abnormalities of uncertain significance. The results of transplantation in this group were then compared with those for similar patients identified from other databases who did not receive high-dose therapy. Prior to transplantation, the majority of patients received salvage chemotherapy, and 62% achieved a response. High-dose chemotherapy consisted of BEAM or alternative chemotherapy-based programs, and approximately one-third received post-transplant radiotherapy. The outcome of transplanted patients (38% versus 29% six-year survival rate) compared favorably with that for conventionally treated patients, but did not achieve statistical significance. Similar to the ASHAP study described above,[28] response to salvage chemotherapy was the only important prognostic factor for overall outcome, and patients who had progressive therapy after second- and third-line therapy had no chance to be cured.

A report from the Autologous Blood and Marrow Transplant Registry identified 122 patients who failed to achieve a complete response after at least one chemotherapy regimen.[38] Inclusion criteria required progressive disease or biopsy confirmation of persistent disease. In this study, 58% of patients received salvage chemotherapy prior to transplant, with 56% of these patients achieving a partial remission. The three-year probabilities of overall and progression-free survival were 50% and 38%, respectively. Although B symptoms and poor performance status were predictors of poor survival, pretransplant chemosensitivity was said not to be a prognostic factor – a finding that is superficially in conflict with the results of Andre et al[37] and Rodriquez et al.[28] However, the conclusion in the current study that chemosensitivity was not predictive of outcome is misleading, since patients who achieved a complete response with second- or third-line therapy were not included in the study group.

A second registry study from the European Group for Bone Marrow Transplantation reviewed the results in a similar group of 175 patients transplanted between 1979 and 1995.[39] In this study, patients were identified as induction failures if they had disease progression or stable disease after primary therapy. Patients who received salvage chemotherapy were excluded if they achieved a response. Data on gallium scans and positron emission tomography (PET) were not included, since they were not routinely performed during the period of study. For this reason, it is possible that some patients who were identified as induction failures may have had residual fibrotic masses without viable tumor, since pathologic confirmation of persistent tumor was not required. With a median follow-up of just over six years, the five-year actuarial overall and progression-free survival rates were 36% and 32%, respectively. The transplant-related mortality rate was 14%. The only factor predictive of survival in a multivariate analysis was a shorter interval between diagnosis and transplant. Although this latter finding suggests that patients should move directly to transplantation once they are identified as induction failures, it is misleading, since patients who achieved a remission with salvage chemotherapy were excluded from the study group.

Taken in summary, the above studies on induction failures provide supportive evidence that approximately one-third of patients can achieve long-term survival following high-dose therapy and stem cell rescue. It is possible that these numbers are somewhat inflated, since some patients who undoubtedly qualified as induction failures did not go on to transplantation because of a decline in performance status associated with disease progression. On the other hand, since the treatment-related mortality rate (8–14% in the above series) is now much lower, overall long-term survival may be improved in current patients with induction failure. One study has suggested that these patients might benefit from tandem courses of high-dose therapy.[40] Nevertheless, it seems unlikely that patients who fail to achieve a response with a modern salvage program are going to benefit from high-dose therapy.

THE ROLE OF GALLIUM AND PET SCANS IN HODGKIN'S DISEASE

As the majority of patients with HD are now treated with systemic therapy, the necessity for precise diagnostic staging has decreased. Thus, the lymphangiogram is currently rarely performed, and most centers have abandoned the staging laparotomy, a procedure that upstages approximately 20% of patients[41] with no radiographic evidence of infradiaphragmatic disease but does not positively impact on survival.[7] In contrast to the lack of enthusiasm for more vigorous diagnostic staging, there is tremendous interest in tests that can determine the viability of residual masses, which are common after treatment of HD. Although the post-therapy gallium scan was until recently considered the best way to distinguish persistent tumor from fibrotic mass, the sensitivity of gallium for detecting small amounts of disease is very limited. For example, Salloum et al[42] studied 101 patients with positive gallium scan at diagnosis, and found that only 4 had a positive post-treatment scan. Two of these four patients had obvious evidence of failure by history, physical examination, or other studies. Of the remaining 97 patients who achieved negative scans, 16 relapsed, including more than one-third of patients with stage III–IV disease. Thus, the post-treatment gallium scan identified only 20% of the patients destined to relapse, and half of these patients were known to have relapse/persistent disease without gallium scan. Similarly, in the same study, no patient had relapse detected by gallium scan prior to computed tomography (CT) or other clinical evidence of disease recurrence. This study suggests that gallium scanning has poor sensitivity for small-volume disease.

More recently, investigators have begun to study the use of early GS (after one or two cycles of chemotherapy), with the theory that a more rapid loss of viability correlates with chemosensitivity and would therefore be more predictive of outcome. Front et al[43] studied 98 patients, of whom 31 had a gallium scan after one cycle of chemotherapy, 83 had a scan after a median of 3.5 cycles, and 16 had scans after one cycle and then at midtreatment. The authors concluded that the results of a gallium scan after one cycle, but not at midtreatment, were predictive of outcome. Of the 31 patients who were scanned after one cycle of treatment, 24 had negative scans, of whom 22 (92%) remained free of disease. In contrast, 4 of the 7 patients with positive scans relapsed or had disease progression. One major problem in this study is that since nearly two-thirds of the patients had early-stage disease and only 10%

had bulky disease, most of the patients would be expected to convert to gallium scan-negativity early after treatment because they had relatively small-volume disease at diagnosis. A better test of the predictive value of an early gallium scan would have been obtained if the study population had been restricted to patients with advanced or bulky disease. Nevertheless, if the predictive value of an early gallium scan is confirmed, it could provide a framework for abbreviating therapy in patients with a quick response or changing therapy in patients who are not responding appropriately. Response-adapted treatment is currently being tested in the ongoing Pediatric Oncology Group (POG) study of early-stage HD (Table 3.1).

Despite the recent enthusiasm for early gallium scanning, mounting evidence suggests that PET imaging with the glucose analog [18F]fluorodeoxyglucose (FDG) will replace gallium scanning and perhaps routine CT and bone marrow biopsies. The major reasons for the potential impact of PET–FDG are that it combines the functional (viability) advantage of the gallium scan with far better image resolution and a sensitivity that compares favorably with that of CT. Unfortunately, analogously to the history of gallium scanning, thus far, most studies of PET imaging have been done after treatment, where even the most exquisite test will fail to detect a small number of tumor cells. Recently, Jerusalem et al[44] studied 54 patients with HD and NHL. Six patients had positive post-treatment scans, all of whom relapsed. However, 5 of 19 patients with negative PET but with residual CT masses relapsed, and 3 patients who were both PET- and CT-negative relapsed. These results are similar to those of post-treatment gallium scanning in that a positive test was accurate in predicting residual disease, while a negative result did not indicate disease sterilization. Zinzani et al[45] recently published more positive data with PET in 44 patients with HD and NHL who presented with abdominal disease. This population of patients was chosen because of the difficulty of gallium-scan interpretation of abdominal disease secondary to nonspecific hepatic uptake and excretion into the bowel. All 13 patients with positive post-treatment scans relapsed, compared with only 1 relapse of 24 patients with a negative post-treatment PET scan. Despite the impressive results of the latter study, it seems likely that the optimal use of PET may be in determining the rate of response, with quickly responding patients presumably having more treatment-sensitive disease. Nevertheless, there are no early PET scan data yet available in patients with HD.

SUMMARY

Advances in molecular biology have unraveled the origin of the Hodgkin's Reed–Sternberg cell, and are providing tremendous insight into HD pathogenesis as well as newer avenues of treatment. Clearly, as gene expression profiles are examined from patients with resistant versus sensitive disease, biological variables will replace surrogate clinical criteria used to recommend treatment. In the meantime, newer imaging studies, especially PET–FDG, may provide a tremendous opportunity to limit therapy in patients with quickly responsive disease or to change therapy in whom viable lymphoma can be identified after one or more cycles of therapy. The enthusiasm for more intensive treatments in patients with advanced disease may bring us back to the age of MOPP when sterility was near-universal in men and age-related in women, and MDS/leukemia was a catastrophic complication of otherwise-successful therapy. Therefore, appropriate patient selection for these trials will represent a challenging problem. Moreover, even if high-dose therapy proves to be superior to regimens such as ABVD, it will also be necessary to prove that it is a better strategy than initial ABVD followed by high-dose therapy for relapsed patients.

REFERENCES

1. Brauninger A, Hansmann ML, Strickler JG et al, Identification of common germinal-center B-cell precursors in two patients with both Hodgkin's disease and non-Hodgkin's lymphoma. N Engl J Med 1999; 340: 1239–47.

2. Marafioti T, Hummel M, Anagnostopoulos I et al, Classical Hodgkin's disease and follicular lymphoma originating from the same germinal center B cell. J Clin Oncol 1999; 17: 3804–9.

3. Kapp U, Yeh WC, Patterson B et al, Inteleukin 13 is secreted by and stimulates the growth of Hodgkin and Reed–Sternberg cells. J Exp Med 1999; 189: 1939–46.

4. Cossman J, Annunziata CM, Barash S et al, Reed–Sternberg cell genome expression supports a B-cell lineage. Blood 1999; 94: 411–16.

5. Hasse U, Tinguely M, Leibundgut EO et al, Clonal loss of heterozygosity in microdissected Hodgkin and Reed–Sternberg cells. J Natl Cancer Inst 1999; 91: 1581–3.

6. Specht L, Gray RG, Clarke MJ, Peto R, Influence of more extensive radiotherapy and adjuvant chemotherapy on long-term outcome of early-stage Hodgkin's disease: a meta-analysis of 23 randomized trials involving 3,888 patients. International Hodgkin's Disease Collaborative Group. J Clin Oncol 1998; 16: 830–43.

7. Carde P, Hagenbeek A, Hayat M et al, Clinical staging versus laparotomy and combined modality with MOPP versus ABVD in early-stage Hodgkin's disease: the H6 twin randomized trials from the European Organization for Research and Treatment of Cancer Lymphoma Cooperative Group. J Clin Oncol 1993; 11: 2258–72.

8. Hagenbeek A, Carde P, Noordijk E et al, Prognostic factor tailored treatment of early stage Hodgkin's disease. Results from a prospective randomized phase III clinical trial in 762 patients (H7 study). Blood 1997; 90(10 Suppl 1): 2603.

9. Wirth A, Chao M, Corry J et al, Mantle irradiation alone for clinical stage I–II Hodgkin's disease: long-term follow-up and analysis of prognostic factors in 261 patients. J Clin Oncol 1999; 17: 230–40.

10. Loeffler M, Diehl V, Pfreundschuh M et al, Dose–response relationship of complementary radiotherapy following four cycles of combination chemotherapy in intermediate-stage Hodgkin's disease. J Clin Oncol 1997; 15: 2275–87.

11. Santoro A, Bonfante V, Viviani S et al, Subtotal nodal vs involved field radiation after 4 cycles of ABVD in early stage Hodgkin's disease. Proc Am Soc Clin Oncol 1996; 15: A1271.

12. Schellong G, The balance between cure and late effects in childhood Hodgkin's lymphoma: the experience of the German–Austrian Study Group since

1978. German–Austrian Pediatric Hodgkin's Disease Study Group. *Ann Oncol* 1996; **7**: 67–72.

13. Salloum E, Doria R, Schubert W et al, Second solid tumors in patients with Hodgkin's disease cured after radiation or chemotherapy plus adjuvant low-dose radiation. *J Clin Oncol* 1996; **14**: 2435–43.

14. Wolden SL, Lamborn KR, Cleary SF et al, Second cancers following pediatric Hodgkin's disease. *J Clin Oncol* 1998; **16**: 536–44.

15. Hancock SL, Tucker MA, Hoppe RT, Factors affecting late mortality from heart disease after treatment of Hodgkin's disease. *JAMA* 1993; **270**: 1949–55.

16. Miettinen M, Franssila KO, Saxen E, Hodgkin's disease, lymphocytic predominance nodular. Increased risk for subsequent non-Hodgkin's lymphomas. *Cancer* 1983; **51**: 2293–300.

17. Diehl V, Sextro M, Franklin J et al, Clinical presentation, course, and prognostic factors in lymphocyte-predominant Hodgkin's disease and lymphocyte-rich classical Hodgkin's disease: report from the European Task Force on Lymphoma Project on Lymphocyte-Predominant Hodgkin's Disease. *J Clin Oncol* 1999; **17**: 776–83.

18. Canellos GP, Anderson JR, Propert KJ et al, Chemotherapy of advanced Hodgkin's disease with MOPP, ABVD, or MOPP alternating with ABVD. *N Engl J Med* 1992; **327**: 1478–84.

19. Connors JM, Klimo P, Adams G et al, treatment of advanced Hodgkin's disease with chemotherapy – comparison of MOPP/ABV hybrid regimen with alternating courses of MOPP and ABVD: a report from the National Cancer Institute of Canada clinical trials group. *J Clin Oncol* 1997; **15**: 1638–45 [erratum 2762].

20. Duggan D, Petroni G, Johnson J et al, MOPP/ABV vs ABVD for advanced Hodgkin's disease: a preliminary report of CALGB 8952 (with SWOG, ECOG, NCIC). *Proc Am Soc Clin Oncol* 1997; **16**: Abst 43.

21. Diehl V, Franklin J, Hasenclever D et al, BEACOPP, a new dose-escalated and accelerated regimen, is at least as effective as COPP/ABVD in patients with advanced-stage Hodgkin's lymphoma: interim report from a trial of the German Hodgkin's Lymphoma Study Group. *J Clin Oncol* 1998; **16**: 3810–21.

22. Tesch H, Diehl V, Lathan B et al, Moderate dose escalation for advanced stage Hodgkin's disease using the bleomycin, etoposide, Adriamycin, cyclophosphamide, vincristine, procarbazine, and prednisone scheme and adjuvant radiotherapy: a study of the German Hodgkin's Lymphoma Study Group. *Blood* 1998; **92**: 4560–7.

23. Carella AM, Prencipe E, Pungolino E et al, Twelve years experience with high-dose therapy and autologous stem cell transplantation for high-risk Hodgkin's disease patients in first remission after MOPP/ABVD chemotherapy. *Leuk Lymphoma* 1996; **21**: 63–70.

24. Hasenclever D, Diehl V, A prognostic score for advanced Hodgkin's disease. International Prognostic Factors Project on Advanced Hodgkin's Disease. *N Engl J Med* 1998; **339**: 1506–14.

25. Sarris AH, Kliche KO, Pethambaram P et al, Interleukin-10 levels are often elevated in serum of adults with Hodgkin's disease and are associated with inferior failure-free survival. *Ann Oncol* 1999; **10**: 433–40.

26. Murray PG, Billingham LJ, Hassan HT et al, Effect of Epstein–Barr virus infection on response to chemotherapy and survival in Hodgkin's disease. *Blood* 1999; **94**: 442–7.

27. Marshall NA, DeVita VT Jr, Hodgkin's disease and transplantation: a room with a (nontransplanter's) view. *Semin Oncol* 1999; **26**: 67–73.

28. Rodriquez J, Rodriquez MA, Fayad L et al, ASHAP: a regimen for cytoreduction of refractory or recurrent Hodgkin's disease. *Blood* 1999; **93**: 3632–6.

29. Aparicio J, Segura A, Garcera S et al, ESHAP is an active regimen for relapsing Hodgkin's disease. *Ann Oncol* 1999; **10**: 593–5.

30. Bonfante V, Viviani S, Santoro A et al, Ifosfamide and vinorelbine: an active regimen for patients with relapsed or refractory Hodgkin's disease. *Br J Haematol* 1998; **103**: 533–5.

31. Brandwein JM, Callum J, Sutcliffe SB et al, Evaluation of cytoreductive therapy prior to high dose treatment with autologous bone marrow transplantation in relapsed and refractory Hodgkin's disease. *Bone Marrow Transplant* 1990; **5**: 99–103.

32. Carrion JR, Garcia Arroyo FR, Salinas P, Infusional chemotherapy (EPOCH) in patients with refractory or relapsed lymphoma. *Am J Clin Oncol* 1995; **18**: 44–6.

33. Harrison CN, Gregory W, Hudson GV et al, High-dose BEAM chemotherapy with autologous haemopoietic stem cell transplantation for Hodgkin's disease is unlikely to be associated with a major increased risk of secondary MDS/AML. *Br J Cancer* 1999; **81**: 476–83.

34. Darrington DL, Vose JM, Anderson JR et al, Incidence and characterization of secondary myelodysplastic syndrome and acute myelogenous leukemia following high-dose chemoradiotherapy and autologous stem-cell transplantation for lymphoid malignancies. *J Clin Oncol* 1994; **12**: 2527–34.

35. Freedman AS, Gribben JG, Neuberg D et al, High-dose therapy and autologous bone marrow transplantation in patients with follicular lymphoma during first remission. *Blood* 1996; **88**: 2780–6.

36. Philip T, Guglielmi C, Hagenbeek A et al, Autologous bone marrow transplantation as compared with salvage chemotherapy in relapses of chemotherapy-sensitive non-Hodgkin's lymphoma. *N Engl J Med* 1995; **333**: 1540–5.

37. Andre M, Henry-Amar M, Pico JL et al, Comparison of high-dose therapy and autologous stem-cell transplantation with conventional therapy for Hodgkin's disease induction failure: a case–control study. Societé Française de Greffe de Moelle. *J Clin Oncol* 1999; **17**: 222–9.

38. Lazarus HM, Rowlings PA, Zhang MJ et al, Autotransplants for Hodgkin's disease in patients never achieving remission: a report from the Autologous Blood and Marrow Transplant Registry. *J Clin Oncol* 1999; **17**: 534–45.

39. Sweetenham JW, Carella AM, Taghipour G et al, High-dose therapy and autologous stem-cell transplantation for adult patients with Hodgkin's disease who do not enter remission after induction chemotherapy: results in 175 patients reported to the European Group for Blood and Marrow Transplantation Lymphoma Working Party. *J Clin Oncol* 1999; **17**: 3101–9.

40. Ahmed T, Lake DE, Beer M et al, Single and double autotransplants for relapsing/refractory Hodgkin's disease: results of two consecutive trials. *Bone Marrow Transplant* 1997; **19**: 449–54.

41. Rueffer U, Sieber M, Josting A et al, Prognostic factors for subdiaphragmatic involvement in clinical stage I–II supra-diaphragmatic Hodgkin's disease: a retrospective analysis of the GHSG. *Ann Oncol* 1999; **10**: 1343–8.

42. Salloum E, Brandt DS, Caride VJ et al, Gallium scans in the management of patients with Hodgkin's disease: a study of 101 patients. *J Clin Oncol* 1997; **15**: 518–27.

43. Front D, Bar-Shalom R, Mor M et al, Hodgkin disease: prediction of outcome with 67 Ga scintigraphy after one cycle of chemotherapy. *Radiology* 1999; **210**: 487–91.

44. Jerusalem G, Beguin Y, Fassotte MF et al, Whole-body positron emission tomography using ^{18}F-fluorodeoxyglucose for posttreatment evaluation in Hodgkin's disease and non-Hodgkin's lymphoma has higher diagnostic and prognostic value than classical computed tomography scan imaging. *Blood* 1999; **94**: 429–33.

45. Zinzani PL, Magagnoli M, Chierichetti F et al, The role of positron emission tomography (PET) in the management of lymphoma patients. *Ann Oncol* 1999; **10**: 1181–4.

4
Follicular lymphomas

Bertrand Coiffier

INTRODUCTION

Follicular lymphoma (FL) is the second most frequent lymphoma, and represents 20–25% of all lymphomas. It is characterized by a proliferation of CD10$^+$ B cells that bear the t(14;18) translocation or *BCL2* gene rearrangement. If the proliferation corresponds initially to small cleaved cells, with time it evolves to larger cells, and this is not always associated with a different outcome. A worse outcome is observed in patients with adverse prognostic parameters exhibiting a large tumor mass, and these patients need to be treated at diagnosis. In population-based series, the median survival is five to six years, which is much shorter than in the usually reported referral center analyses. The only regimen associated with a survival improvement in comparative trials for patients with adverse parameters consists of an interferon-α together with or following a doxorubicin-containing regimen. This may change when the results of randomized studies incorporating monoclonal antibodies become known. After one or several relapses, sometimes at the time of diagnosis, the disease transforms into a more aggressive lymphoma characterized by a proliferation of large non-cleaved cells or Burkitt-like cells. At this time, patients usually have a large tumor mass, B symptoms, and high lactate dehydrogenase (LDH) level. The duration of the response to any treatment is short except for patients treated with high-dose therapy and autologous stem cell transplantation. This treatment was also used in first relapse, and seems to be associated with a better outcome than standard chemotherapy, even though no comparative study has been reported. This benefit is particularly true for patients where a clearance of *BCL2*-rearranged cells was observed. During the year 1999, some of these points were emphasized or developed.

CLASSIFICATION

Sometimes patients present different aspects of the lymphoma either in the same tumor or in different tumors. This type of lymphoma is called 'composite lymphoma' in the World Health Organization classification.[1,2] However, this term may cover different abnormalities, mostly resulting from diagnosis being made at a time when the follicular lymphoma is already in transformation into a more aggressive lymphoma in some parts of the tumor. This may be called a transformed FL at diagnosis, but it is not completely certain that it bears the adverse outcome associated with secondary transformations in FL. More rarely, the lymphoma associates two types of indolent lymphomas, for example FL and mantle cell lymphoma (MCL), FL and marginal zone lymphoma (MZL), or FL and Hodgkin's lymphoma. It is not completely clear whether this situation represent two different diseases or a different molecular evolution of the same lymphoma. Results of fine-tuned molecular analyses presented in 1999 are compatible with both hypotheses. Aiello et al[3] presented one patient with FL and mucosa-associated lymphoid tissue (MALT) lymphomas in whom the polymerase chain reaction (PCR) analysis of the rearranged immunoglobulin heavy-chain gene, the t(14;18) translocation, and CDR3 sequence from each lesion indicated a common clonal lineage. Brauninger et al[4] and Marafioti et al[5] presented three patients with Hodgkin's and non-Hodgkin's B-cell lymphoma. In these patients, the Reed–Sternberg cells were related clonally to the non-Hodgkin's lymphoma B cells. In contrast, Fend et al[6] described the detailed immunohistochemical and molecular findings in three cases with features of composite low-grade B-cell lymphoma. Sequence analysis of isolated cell populations revealed unrelated clonal rearrangements in each of the two tumor parts in all three cases, suggesting distinct clonal origins.

In some patients, the final diagnosis of the lymphoma type may be difficult. In some FL cases, this may only be done if the t(14;18) is demonstrated, but this translocation is not present or demonstrable in all cases. The BCL6 protein that is expressed mainly by follicle center cells and a few interfollicular T lymphocytes may be of some help. Raible et al[7] analyzed BCL6 expression as an aid to differentiation of tumors with follicle center origin in 72 indolent lymphomas. All of 31 FL cases were positive for BCL6 expression. One of 13 small lymphocytic lymphoma (SLL) cases and 1 of 12 MCL cases were positive, whereas none of 16 MZL cases was positive.

PROGNOSTIC PARAMETERS

Although standard prognostic parameters have been described and recognized by the whole community for aggressive lymphomas,[8] such prognostic parameters have not been identified in FL patients. The Groupe d'Etude des Lymphomes de l'Adulte (GELA) has described its observations.[9] Their analysis included 484 patients with stage III–IV treated in two phase III trials. Poor prognostic factors for overall survival in univariate analyses were age over 60 years, B symptoms, more than one extranodal site, stage IV, tumor bulk greater than 7 cm, at least three nodal sites larger than 3 cm, liver involvement, serous effusion compression or orbital/epidural involvement, and erythrocyte sedimentation rate greater than 30 mm. In a multivariate analysis, three factors remained significant: B symptoms (risk ratio = 1.80), age over 60 years (risk ratio = 1.60), and at least three nodal sites larger than 3 cm (risk ratio = 1.71). When the International Prognostic Index (IPI) was applied to these patients, the numbers of patients with scores 0–1, 2, 3, and 4–5 were 49%, 39%, 11%, and 2%, respectively, and this index was significantly associated with progression-free survival ($p = 0.002$) and overall survival ($p = 0.0001$). However, the number of patients in high-risk groups was low. To isolate a group of patients requiring a more aggressive therapy, the IPI is not the best index, and an international collaborative study is currently running to describe a better one.

Bechter et al[10] have shown in a retrospective study that the strong expression of LFA-1 (CD11a, CD18) on FL cells is associated with a longer survival compared with patients with a weak or moderate expression of both antigens. Furthermore, a multivariate analysis identified CD18 as a new independent prognostic factor in patients with advanced FL. However, the number of patients and biologic parameters included in this analysis were too low to allow definitive conclusions to be drawn regarding the significance of this adhesion molecule.

Tezcan et al[11] evaluated the outcome and prognostic factors of 40 patients with localized stage FL treated by the Nebraska Lymphoma Study Group. The follicular large cell type represented 75% of the cases, and in 14 of them it existed as a diffuse component. The initial treatment was radiation therapy to the involved field in 15 patients, anthracycline-containing chemotherapy in 20, and combined-modality treatment in 5. The median follow-up was 10 years. Of the 37 patients achieving complete remission (CR), only 7 were alive in first CR, 1 died owing to sepsis, another died because of a myeloproliferative disorder at 77 months following chemotherapy, and 6 died in first CR because of unrelated causes. Twenty-two patients relapsed between 1 and 128 months following the CR. The estimated 10-year event-free survival and overall survival rates were 21% and 44%, respectively. Various factors, including histologic subtype, stage, and degree of follicularity, did not influence the outcome. This study showed a high recurrence rate, and chemotherapy seems to be associated with a better outcome. However, it did not confirm that some patients with localized FL may be cured.

Wood et al[12] described the outcome of advanced-stage FL patients based on a population-based cohort observed in Alberta, Canada. Approximately 45% of the 157 patients had died at last follow-up. Treatment was initiated at the time of diagnosis in 87 patients (55%), with alkylating agents used in 66% of them. Of the 70 patients not treated at initial diagnosis, 69% had been treated at a median of 16.3 months. The overall median survival was 5.9 years. By multivariate analysis, the only factors that influenced survival were LDH level and B symptoms. An elevated LDH level had a hazard ratio of 2.8 and a median survival of 8.0 years versus 3.6 years ($p < 0.0001$). B symptoms had a hazard ratio of 2.3 and a median survival of 6.5 years versus 3.1 years ($p < 0.01$). The median overall survival of 5.9 years was worse than in previous non-population-based reports. This study is probably a better reflection of reality than studies conducted in referral centers, and it clearly emphasizes that a large group of FL patients have a poor outcome.

For years, it was debated whether follicular lymphoma with a large cell component has a clinical behavior distinct from other FL. Rodriguez et al[13] reported 100 patients treated at the MD Anderson Cancer Center within three successive programs. With a median follow-up of 67 months, the five-year survival rate was 72% and the failure-free survival rate 67%. As Rodriguez et al found that these patients had clinical features, prognostic factors, and response to treatment similar to those reported for diffuse large cell lymphoma, they concluded that this lymphoma is an aggressive one and should be treated like diffuse large cell lymphoma. This conclusion should only have been drawn if patients with large cell FL had been compared with patients with small cell or mixed FL. This has never been done in the USA. However, in large-scale retrospective analyses such as the one conducted by Armitage and colleagues,[14,15] the survival of FL patients was identical whatever the percentage of large cells. Moreover, in a randomized trial, patients with grade 3 FL had a survival similar to those with grade 2 FL, both worse than the survival of grade 1 FL patients.[16] Thus, the conviction of American authors that FL with a large cell component must be considered as an aggressive lymphoma has never been confirmed in any prospective trial, and we continue to recommend that FL patients must be allocated to different treatments on the basis of the presence or absence of adverse prognostic parameters but not on the fact that there exists a proliferation with large cells in some parts of the lymph nodes. The very good survival found in this study compared with that found in the previously reported population-based analysis[12] confirms the selection bias regularly found in American referral centers.

TREATMENT

The t(14;18) translocation is the landmark of follicular lymphoma, and, with the improvement of molecular techniques, it may be found in nearly 100% of patients, even if the classical *BCL2* gene rearrangement is only found in 60–70% of cases. The disappearance of cells with *BCL2* rearrangement from blood or bone marrow was associated with a better outcome in several studies. However, false-positive and false-negative results may be observed in some studies, and up to now no standard validation procedure has been described to validate the results. Johnson et al[17] have conducted a collaborative study to test the reliability of PCR and to compare results from different laboratories in Europe and North America. Twenty laboratories were sent blood from normal donors with varying numbers of t(14;18)-bearing cells added from a cell line with a translocation in the major breakpoint region of the *BCL2* gene. The false-positive rate was 28%, with 11 samples from 9 laboratories reported as positive when no t(14;18) cells were added. They concluded that the PCR to detect *BCL2–IgH* rearrangements is presently carried out with widely disparate results. Further effort is required to develop a standard PCR protocol that can be re-tested in different laboratories to improve accuracy and reproducibility. Until this standardization has been done, it is probably difficult or impossible to base a therapeutic decision on the results of *BCL2* gene rearrangement detection by PCR.

Standard chemotherapy

Coiffier et al[16] reported a study from the GELA in elderly patients with high-risk FL. Patients over 60 years old with an adverse prognosis defined by the presence of a large tumor mass, poor performance status, B symptoms, above-normal LDH level, or a β_2-microglobulin level of 3 mg/l or more were randomized between CHVP (cyclophosphamide 600 mg/m^2, doxorubicin 25 mg/m^2, teniposide 60 mg/m^2, and prednisone 40 mg/m^2 × 5 days, given in 12 cycles in 18 months) plus interferon-α (IFN-α) (5 MU three times a week for 18 months) or fludarabine alone (25 mg/m^2/day × 5 days for 6 cycles, then 20 mg/m^2/day for 6 further cycles for 18 months). Patients treated with CHVP plus IFN-α had a greater response to treatment, a longer time to progression, and a longer survival than those treated with fludarabine alone ($p < 0.05$) for all analyses). With a median follow-up of 29 months, the two-year failure-free survival rate was 63% for the CHVP plus IFN-α arm compared with 49% for the fludarabine arm, while the two-year survival rates were 77% and 62%, respectively. This benefit was confirmed in a multivariate analysis including initial prognostic parameters. Fludarabine alone was associated with less neutropenia than CHVP plus IFN-α. IFN-α was decreased or stopped in 39% of the patients because of severe fatigue. In this randomized study, patients were older than in the first trial,[18] thus, they tolerated the IFN-α less well, with more patients stopping it before the end of the scheduled treatment. However, even with this early stopping, survival and event-free survival were longer than in the fludarabine arm. Fludarabine alone is insufficient to give good responses and long survivals in patients with aggressive disease. Combinations of fludarabine with other drugs such as mitoxantrone or cyclophosphamide plus corticosteroids have been associated with better results in phase II studies,[19,20] but these combinations have not been tested in a comparative trial. Their hematologic toxicity may be greater than with a doxorubicin-containing regimen.[20] Up to now, the combination of CHVP and IFN-α is the only treatment that has been associated with a better survival in any comparative study.

Another purine analog, cladribine, was tested in a phase II trial in 55 patients.[21] Survival and event-free survival were comparable to those observed with fludarabine alone in the previous trial. Several other small phase II trials[22] have shown that fludarabine or cladribine alone are associated with few toxic events and are very well tolerated, but their efficacy is always lower than a doxorubicin-containing regimen. There is no justification for including patients in such trials or for using these drugs alone in first-line patients where the main objective of the treatment must be to reach as long a survival as possible. These drugs may have a better efficacy if they are combined with other active drugs, but this should only be tested in randomized trials. Until the results of such studies are available, they should only be used in relapsing patients.

A retrospective analysis of patients with stage I or II disease treated with radiotherapy as initial treatment has been presented.[23] All patients were analyzed, whatever the type of lymphoma. However, a sufficient number of patients with FL was included to allow the conclusion that radiotherapy alone may be associated with very good local control of the disease but that it relapsed outside the initial site. The results were slightly better when radiotherapy was combined with chemotherapy. The place of the radiotherapy has not yet been completely defined yet, and probably never will be. It certainly has a role to play in elderly patients with localized disease. For young patients, it may only be associated with local control for a few years.

Several combinations have been presented for relapsing patients. For those who are scheduled for high-dose therapy and autologous stem cell transplantation, the best regimen is a non-toxic one with an overall response rate greater than 70%. Few regimens satisfy these criteria. The IAPVP-16 regimen (ifosfamide 5 g/m^2 on day 1, etoposide 100 mg/m^2 on days 1–3, cytarabine 1.2 g/m^2/12 hours on days 1 and 2, and methylprednisolone 80 mg/m^2 on days 1–5)[24] has a 80% response rate, but has been associated with severe neutropenia and thrombocytopenia in at least two-thirds of patients. Nevertheless, it seems to be possible to harvest hematopoietic stem cells for an autotransplant in most patients. Combinations with purine analogs are often associated with a severe hematologic toxicity, and are not recommended in multitreated patients or for those scheduled for autologous transplantation.[25,26]

Monoclonal antibody treatment

Over the past few years, several studies have reported the activity of rituximab (Mabthera, Rituxan), a chimeric monoclonal anti-CD20 antibody, in FL and other lymphomas.[27–29] During 1999, several reports gave complementary information on this activity.[30–32] In relapsing FL, a response rate greater than 50% (complete or partial) was obtained in 50–65% of patients, even in those refractory to previous treatment, those previously treated with high-dose therapy, or those with bulky tumors.[33] These response rates were lower in other lymphomas. The duration of response was about one year. Rarely patients relapsed with CD20$^-$ cells, showing clonal selection by the antibody therapy.[34]

In another trial, the standard dose of rituximab (375 mg/m^2/week for 4 weeks) was extended to 8 weeks in a small group of patients.[35] The toxicity and response rate did not seem to be different from those with the standard treatment. Even though the duration of the response seems a little longer, it is not yet appropriate to modify the standard use of this drug. This can only be done after a randomized comparison of the two schedules has been performed.

Czuczman[36] reported a combination of CHOP (cyclophosphamide, doxorubicin, vincristine, and prednisone) and rituximab in previously untreated patients with FL. Forty patients with low-grade or follicular B-cell lymphoma received six infusions of rituximab (375 mg/m^2) in combination with six cycles of CHOP chemotherapy. The overall response rate was 95%. Twenty-two patients experienced a complete response (55%), 16 had a partial response (40%), and two who did not receive the planned treatment were classified as non-responders. Medians for duration of response and time to progression had not been reached after a median observation of 29 months. Twenty-eight of 38 assessable patients (74%) are still in remission. The observed toxicity was not cumulative compared with what was expected from CHOP or rituximab alone. The *BCL2* gene was rearranged in eight patients; seven of these reached a complete remission and converted to a molecular remission by completion of therapy. These particularly interesting results should have already been confirmed in a comparative trial with or without rituximab. Such a trial is not even ongoing at the time of this review. However, only such a trial may definitively settle the place of this interesting drug in our armamentarium for FL patients.

A severe toxicity was described in patients with high blood involvement at time of treatment, mostly patients with chronic lymphocytic leukemia or MCL.[37–39] This syndrome related to acute cytosis of circulating lymphoma cells, and secondary secretion of cytokines was rarely observed in FL patients.

Monoclonal mouse anti-CD20 antibody radiolabeled with iodine-131 (^{131}I) (tositumomab, Bexxar) given at non-myeloablative doses yield remissions in 75–80% of cases, including 35–40% complete remissions.[40,41] High-dose ^{131}I-anti-B1 antibody with stem cell transplantation generates objective responses in 85–90% of cases, including 75–80% complete remissions.[42] Although more patients need to be evaluated with a longer follow-up period and in control studies, radioimmunotherapy appears to be an effective and well-tolerated treatment. In 1999, updates of previous trials with ^{131}I-anti-CD20 antibody presented complementary information.

Wiseman et al[43] presented the first results for another mouse monoclonal antibody labeled with yttrium-90 (^{90}Y). Ibritumomab, the murine counterpart to rituximab, radiolabeled with ^{90}Y (Zevalin), gave an overall response rate of 64% or 67% in two phase I studies. Witzig et al[44] reported the results of a phase I/II trial with ibritumomab, conducted to determine the maximum tolerated single dose that could be administered without stem cell support and to evaluate safety and efficacy. Eligible patients had relapsed or refractory CD20$^+$ B-cell lymphoma. The maximum tolerated dose was 0.4 mCi/kg (0.3 mCi/kg for patients with baseline platelet counts of 100 000–149 000/μl). The overall response rate for the intent-to-treat population ($n = 51$) was 67% (26% complete and 41% partial) and for indolent lymphomas ($n = 34$), 82% (26% complete and 56% partial). The duration of response was one year. Adverse events were primarily hematologic, and correlated with baseline extent of bone marrow involvement and baseline platelet count. These results were not so different from those obtained with the ^{131}I-labeled antibody.

These two radiolabeled antibodies gave very interesting results in phase II studies, but their use is more complicated than rituximab treatment. Moreover, no randomized studies comparing these drugs with rituximab or with standard therapies have been presented. Thus, although these drugs might have an important role in the future, this has yet to be proven. As they are more expensive and potentially more toxic than rituximab or standard regimens, any recommendation for their use can only be derived from such comparative studies.

High-dose therapy with transplantation

High-dose therapy (HDT) with autologous stem cell transplantation may be associated with a longer disease-free survival in patients treated in first- or second-line progression, but this has not yet been fully demonstrated in a comparative study. In large single-center trials, it seems to be associated with a longer time to next progression than that observed with standard therapy used in first or second line. An update of the patients treated in the Dana Farber Cancer Institute has been presented by Freedman et al.[45] All 153 patients with relapsed FL were treated with high-dose cyclophosphamide, total-body irradiation, and anti-B-cell monoclonal antibody-purged autologous bone marrow transplantation (ABMT). All patients had received multiple chemotherapy regimens before ABMT, and overt bone marrow infiltration was present in 47% of them at the time of transplant. The disease-free and overall survival rates were estimated to be 42% and 66% at eight years, respectively. Patients whose harvested stem cells were negative by PCR for BCL2–IgH rearrangement after purging experienced longer freedom from recurrence than those whose harvested cells remained PCR-positive ($p < 0.0001$). The fact that follow-up bone marrow samples stayed PCR-negative was strongly predictive of a continued complete response. Although these results strongly recommend HDT in first relapse, they did not demonstrate that purged autologous bone marrow cells are the best harvest. Similar results in term of disease-free and overall survival have been obtained with unpurged peripheral blood stem cells.[46]

FL in transformation is a very aggressive disease, and although patients may respond to standard therapy, time to next progression and survival after the histologic transformation is usually shorter than one year. Selected patients with histologic transformation, particularly those whose transformation occurs early in the course of their disease and who remain chemosensitive, may experience prolonged survival after HDT.[47]

Apostolidis et al[48] have presented the pattern of recurrence and survival after recurrence in FL patients treated with HDT. They reviewed 99 patients treated with cyclophosphamide, total-body irradiation, and ABMT as consolidation of second or subsequent remission. The median length of follow-up was 5.5 years, and 33 patients (33%) developed recurrent lymphoma a median of 14 months after HDT. In 26 patients, the recurrence was detected by the patient, but in 7 it was detected on surveillance investigation. Twenty-six patients presented with recurrence in previous sites of disease. Twenty-two patients (67%)

had FL at the time of recurrence, but in 11 (33%), there was evidence of transformation into diffuse large B-cell lymphoma. Out of the eight patients managed expectantly, five were alive 21–53 months later. Twenty-five patients have required treatment; eight remained alive 6 months to 10 years later, and five were in remission. The five-year survival rate was estimated as 45% (95% confidence interval 27–62%). Survival after recurrence and overall survival after diagnosis were similar to those of historical control group who received conventional treatment (adjusted hazard ratio (HR) = 1.56, p = 0.3, and HR = 1.34, p = 0.4, respectively). These results suggest that HDT at time of second response does not compromise outcome in patients in whom it fails.

Until recently, BCL2-rearranged cells persisted in blood and bone marrow of FL patients, and this persistence may be related to the recurrence of lymphoma after HDT. Trials with ex vivo purging and selection of CD34[+] cells were not convincing, because they only resulted in a few logs decrease of the BCL2-rearranged cells.[49,50] It has been demonstrated that the clinical response to rituximab therapy in FL patients was associated with a clearance of the BCL rearranged cells in blood and bone marrow, even for patients in partial remission with persisting increased lymph nodes. Thus, stem cell harvest after rituximab therapy may collect purer hematopoietic stem cells without or with less detectable BCL2-rearranged cells. Several abstracts were presented during the last American Society of Hematology meeting, with preliminary results demonstrating this possibility.[51] Buckstein et al[52] administered rituximab to 10 patients two days before the harvest. In these patients, the number of harvested CD34[+] cells was identical to those in historic controls, and the duration of neutropenia or thrombocytopenia after HDT was not increased. However, no results have yet been presented for the relapse rate after this treatment, and the efficacy of one injection of rituximab two days before the harvest may be questioned. Several other modalities of rituximab administration are currently being tested, but the administration of the classical four-week treatment some weeks before the harvest may be more interesting because of the long half-life of rituximab and the delay to reach the best response that have been described in previous studies.[27,28]

Allogeneic transplantation may have the advantages over autologous transplant of inducing a graft-versus-lymphoma effect in combination with the killing of lymphoma cells by high-dose chemotherapy. Its use is prevented by its higher toxicity profile. Few studies have tried to compare both modalities. Verdonck[53] reported a small study conducted to compare the results of myeloablative therapy followed either by autologous stem cell transplantation (SCT) or allogeneic SCT for poor-risk low-grade lymphoma. Eighteen patients received autologous SCT and 15 received allogeneic SCT. All autologous transplant patients had chemosensitive disease, while this was the case in only eight of the allogeneic transplant patients. Despite this unfavorable characteristic, all allogeneic transplant patients achieved complete remission with this procedure, and, so far none has relapsed. In contrast, 14 of 18 autologous transplant patients achieved complete remission with SCT and 11 (79%) relapsed. Four allogeneic transplant patients (27%) died from treatment-related complications, whereas none did so with autologous SCT. The three-year probabilities of relapse, overall survival, and event-free survival were 0%, 70%, and 70%, respectively, for allogeneic SCT, and 78%, 33%, and 22%, respectively, for autologous SCT. The differences in relapse and event-free survival were highly significant. However, this was not a randomized study but a retrospective analysis, and the low number of patients may have introduced a lot of biases between the two groups. Moreover, the results for the autologous transplant group were much worse than those published by other investigators. This may be secondary to the fact that this treatment was used late in the disease for patients who had received several previous treatments.

Other therapeutic modalities

Vaccination against lymphoma cells is a promising new developed treatment. The patient's lymphoma cells are used to construct a vaccine including an adjuvant such as granulocyte–macrophage colony-stimulating factor (GM-CSF) or a toxin. The first clinical efficacy of such a therapy was reported by Bendandi et al.[54] They evaluated the ability of a new idiotype protein vaccine to eradicate residual BCL2[+] lymphoma cells in 11 patients in first clinical complete remission after chemotherapy. All 11 patients had BCL2[+] cells detectable in their blood both at diagnosis and after chemotherapy. Eight of these patients had a disappearance of BCL2[+] cells in their blood after vaccination, and sustained their molecular remission during the short reported follow-up. Vaccination allows the clearance of residual tumor cells from blood, and it may be associated with a long disease-free survival. Two other groups are working on this promising therapeutic modality, but it is presently quite expensive and time-consuming, preventing its administration on a large-scale basis or in a randomized trial.

Antisense oligonucleotides have the ability to selectively block disease-causing genes, thereby inhibiting production of disease-associated proteins. Targeting the initiating codon of the BCL2 gene decreases both cell viability and BCL2 protein expression in FL cell lines that overexpress BCL2. An update of a phase I clinical study and several reviews of this modality were reported in 1999.[55–57] Evidence of efficacy includes a responder with stage IV follicular lymphoma who achieved complete clinical and radiologic response that has lasted for more than two years. Other antisense reagents are also in development. In the future, antisense therapy followed by chemotherapy may overcome chemoresistance, to provide effective therapy for a range of malignancies.

BRIEF SUMMARY CONCERNING POSSIBLE DEVELOPMENTS

FL continues to be a model among lymphomas because of the BCL2 rearrangement and the possibility of using this as a marker. The quantitative methods recently developed will allow more precise studies correlating the outcome of different treatment and the level of *BCL2*-rearranged cells in blood or bone marrow. However, careful attention needs to be paid to the accuracy of this technique and its reproducibility among different laboratories.

Monoclonal antibodies are definitely an improvement in the treatment of these patients, but their full role has not been settled. Comparative studies incorporating these agents in different strategies are recommended. Patients' cure rate will probably increase if these agents are well used, but without randomized trials, we may fail to find the best approach. This will be the case for vaccines and antisense drugs too, if they are developed.

REFERENCES

1. Harris NL, Jaffe ES, Diebold J et al, World Health Organization Classification of Neoplastic Diseases of the Hematopoietic and Lymphoid Tissues: Report of the Clinical Advisory Committee Meeting, Airlie House, Virginia, November 1997. *J Clin Oncol* 1999; **17**: 3835–49.

2. Jaffe ES, Harris NL, Diebold J et al, World Health Organization classification of neoplastic diseases of the hematopoietic and lymphoid tissues: a progress report. *Am J Clin Pathol* 1999; **111**: S8–12.

3. Aiello A, Du MQ, Diss TC et al, Simultaneous phenotypically distinct but clonally identical mucosa-associated lymphoid tissue and follicular lymphoma in a patient with Sjögren's syndrome. *Blood* 1999; **94**: 2247–51.

4. Brauninger A, Hansmann ML, Strickler JG et al, Identification of common germinal-center B-cell precursors in two patients with both Hodgkin's disease and non-Hodgkin's lymphoma. *N Engl J Med* 1999; **340**: 1239–47.

5. Marafioti T, Hummel M, Anagnostopoulos I et al, Classical Hodgkin's disease and follicular lymphoma originating from the same germinal center B cell. *J Clin Oncol* 1999; **17**: 3804–9.

6. Fend F, Quintanilla-Martinez L, Kumar S et al, Composite low grade B-cell lymphomas with two immunophenotypically distinct cell populations are true biclonal lymphomas: a molecular analysis using laser capture microdissection. *Am J Pathol* 1999; **154**: 1857–66.

7. Raible MD, Hsi ED, Alkan S, Bcl-6 protein expression by follicle center lymphomas: a marker for differentiating follicle center lymphomas from other low-grade lymphoproliferative disorders. *Am J Clin Pathol* 1999; **112**: 101–7.

8. The International Non-Hodgkin's Lymphoma Prognostic Factors Project, A predictive model for aggressive non-Hodgkin's lymphoma. *N Engl J Med* 1993; **329**: 987–94.

9. Decaudin D, Lepage E, Brousse N et al, Low-grade stage III–IV follicular lymphoma: multivariate analysis of prognostic factors in 484 patients – a study of the Groupe d'Etude des Lymphomes de l'Adulte. *J Clin Oncol* 1999; **17**: 2499–505.

10. Bechter OE, Eisterer W, Dirnhofer S, et al, Expression of LFA-1 identifies different prognostic subgroups in patients with advance follicle center lymphoma (FCL). *Leuk Res* 1999; **23**: 483–8.

11. Tezcan H, Vose JM, Bast M et al, Limited stage I and II follicular non-Hodgkin's lymphoma: the Nebraska Lymphoma Study Group experience. *Leuk Lymphoma* 1999; **34**: 273–85.

12. Wood LA, Coupland RW, North SA et al, Outcome of advanced stage low grade follicular lymphomas in a population-based retrospective cohort. *Cancer* 1999; **85**: 1361–8.

13. Rodriguez J, McLaughlin P, Hagemeister FB et al, Follicular large cell lymphoma: an aggressive lymphoma that often presents with favorable prognostic features. *Blood* 1999; **93**: 2202–7.

14. Armitage JO, Weisenburger DD, New approach to classifying non-Hodgkin's lymphomas: clinical features of the major histologic subtypes. *J Clin Oncol* 1998; **16**: 2780–95.

15. The Non-Hodgkin's Lymphoma Classification Project, A clinical trial of the International Lymphoma Study Group classification of non-Hodgkin's lymphoma. *Blood* 1997; **89**: 3909–18.

16. Coiffier B, Neidhardt-Berard EM, Tilly H et al, Fludarabine alone compared to CHVP plus interferon in elderly patients with follicular lymphoma and adverse prognostic parameters: a GELA study. *Ann Oncol* 1999; **10**: 1191–7.

17. Johnson PW, Swinbank K, MacLennan S et al, Variability of polymerase chain reaction detection of the bcl-2–IgH translocation in an international multicentre study. *Ann Oncol* 1999; **10**: 1349–54.

18. Solal-Celigny P, Lepage E, Brousse N et al, Recombinant interferon alfa-2b combined with a regimen containing doxorubicin in advanced follicular lymphoma. *N Engl J Med* 1993; **329**: 1608–14.

19. McLaughlin P, Hagemeister FB, Romaguera JE et al, Fludarabine, mitoxantrone, and dexamethasone: an effective new regimen for indolent lymphoma. *J Clin Oncol* 1996; **14**: 1262–8.

20. Lazzarino R, Orlandi E, Montillo M et al, Fludarabine, cyclophosphamide, and dexamethasone (FluCyD) combination is effective in pretreated low-grade non-Hodgkin's lymphoma. *Ann Oncol* 1999; **10**: 59–64.

21. Fridrik MA, Jager G, Kienzer HR et al, Efficacy and toxicity of 2-chlorodeoxyadenosine (cladribine), 2 h infusion for 5 days, as first-line treatment for advanced low grade non-Hodgkin's lymphoma. *Eur J Cancer* 1998; **34**: 1560–4.

22. Laurencet FM, Zulian GB, Guetty-Alberto M et al, Cladribine with cyclophosphamide and prednisone in the management of low-grade lymphoproliferative malignancies. *Br J Cancer* 1999; **79**: 1215–19.

23. Kamath SS, Marcus RB, Lynch JW et al, The impact of radiotherapy dose and other treatment-related and clinical factors on in-field control in stage I and II non-Hodgkin's lymphoma. *Int J Radiat Oncol Biol Phys* 1999; **44**: 563–8.

24. Lopez R, Martino R, Brunet S et al, Salvage chemotherapy with IAPVP-16 for advanced refractory or relapsed follicular lymphomas. *Haematologica* 1999; **84**: 911–16.

25. Robak T, Gora-Tybor J, Urbanska-Rys H et al, Combination regimen of 2-chlorodeoxyadenosine (cladribine), mitoxantrone and dexamethasone (CMD) in the treatment of refractory and recurrent low grade non-Hodgkin's lymphoma. *Leuk Lymphoma* 1999; **32**: 359–63.

26. Micallef INM, Lillington DM, Apostolidis J et al, Therapy-related myelodysplasia and secondary acute myelogenous leukemia after high-dose therapy with autologous hematopoietic progenitor-cell support for lymphoid malignancies. *J Clin Oncol* 2000; **18**: 947–55.

27. Maloney D, Grillo-López A, White C et al, IDEC-C2B8 (rituximab) anti-CD20 monoclonal antibody therapy in patients with relapsed low-grade non-Hodgkin's lymphoma. *Blood* 1997; **90**: 2188–95.

28. McLaughlin P, Grillo-Lopez AJ, Link BK et al, Rituximab chimeric anti-CD20 monoclonal antibody therapy for relapsed indolent lymphoma: half of patients respond to a four-dose treatment program. *J Clin Oncol* 1998; **16**: 2825–33.

29. Coiffier B, Haioun C, Ketterer N et al, Rituximab (anti-CD20 monoclonal antibody) for the treatment of patients with relapsing or refractory aggressive lymphoma. A multicenter phase II study. *Blood* 1998; **92**: 1927–32.

30. Grillo-Lopez AJ, White CA, Varns C et al, Overview of the clinical development of rituximab: first monoclonal anti-

body approved for the treatment of lymphoma. *Semin Oncol* 1999; **26**: 66–73.

31. McLaughlin P, Hagemeister FB, Grillo-Lopez AJ, Rituximab in indolent lymphoma: the single-agent pivotal trial. *Semin Oncol* 1999; **26**: 79–87.

32. Berinstein NL, Grillo-Lopez AJ, White CA et al, Association of serum rituximab (IDEC-C2B8) concentration and anti-tumor response in the treatment of recurrent low-grade or follicular non-Hodgkin's lymphoma. *Ann Oncol* 1998; **9**: 995–1001.

33. Davis TA, White CA, Grillo-Lopez AJ et al, Single-agent monoclonal antibody efficacy in bulky non-Hodgkin's lymphoma: results of a phase II trial of rituximab. *J Clin Oncol* 1999; **17**: 1851–7.

34. Schmitz K, Brugger W, Weiss B et al, Clonal selection of CD20-negative non-Hodgkin's lymphoma cells after treatment with anti-CD20 antibody rituximab. *Br J Haematol* 1999; **106**: 571–2.

35. Piro LD, White CA, Grillo-Lopez AJ et al, extended rituximab (anti-CD20 monoclonal antibody) therapy for relapsed or refractory low-grade or follicular non-Hodgkin's lymphoma. *Ann Oncol* 1999; **10**: 655–61.

36. Czuczman MS, CHOP plus rituximab chemoimmunotherapy of indolent B-cell lymphoma. *Semin Oncol* 1999; **26**: 88–96.

37. Byrd JC, Waselenko JK, Maneatis TJ et al, Rituximab therapy in hematologic malignancy patients with circulating blood tumor cells: association with increased infusion-related side effects and rapid blood tumor clearance. *J Clin Oncol* 1999; **17**: 791–5.

38. Yang H, Rosove MH, Figlin RA, Tumor lysis syndrome occurring after the administration of rituximab in lymphoproliferative disorders: high-grade non-Hodgkin's lymphoma and chronic lymphocytic leukemia. *Am J Hematol* 1999; **62**: 247–50.

39. Winkler U, Jensen M, Manzke O et al, Cytokine-release syndrome in patients with B-cell chronic lymphocytic leukemia and high lymphocyte counts after treatment with an anti-CD20 mono-clonal antibody (rituximab, IDEC-C2B8). *Blood* 1999; **94**: 2217–24.

40. Press OW, Eary JF, Appelbaum FR et al, Phase II trial of I-131-B1 (anti-CD20) antibody therapy with autologous stem cell transplantation for relapsed B cell lymphomas. *Lancet* 1995; **346**: 336–40.

41. Kaminski MS, Zelenetz AD, Press O et al, Multicenter phase III study of iodine-131 tositumomab (anti-B1 antibody) for chemotherapy-refractory low-grade or transformed low-grade non-Hodgkin's lymphoma. *Blood* 1998; **92**: 316a.

42. Liu SY, Eary JF, Petersdorf SH et al, Follow-up of relapsed B-cell lymphoma patients treated with iodine-131-labeled anti-CD20 antibody and autologous stem-cell rescue. *J Clin Oncol* 1998; **16**: 3270–8.

43. Wiseman GA, White CA, Witzig TE et al, Radioimmunotherapy of relapsed non-Hodgkin's lymphoma with zevalin, a 90Y-labeled anti-CD20 monoclonal antibody. *Clin Cancer Res* 1999; **5**: 3281s–6s.

44. Witzig TE, White CA, Wiseman GA et al, Phase I/II trial of IDEC-Y2B8 radioimmunotherapy for treatment of relapsed or refractory CD20+ B-cell non-Hodgkin's lymphoma. *J Clin Oncol* 1999; **17**: 3793–803.

45. Freedman AS, Neuberg D, Mauch P et al, Long-term follow-up of autologous bone marrow transplantation in patients with relapsed follicular lymphoma. *Blood* 1999; **94**: 3325–33.

46. Lopez R, Martino R, Sureda A et al, Autologous stem cell transplantation in advanced follicular lymphoma. A single center experience. *Haematologica* 1999; **84**: 350–5.

47. Friedberg JW, Neuberg D, Gribben JG et al, Autologous bone marrow transplantation after histologic transformation of indolent B cell malignancies. *Biol Blood Marrow Transplant* 1999; **5**: 262–8.

48. Apostolidis J, Foran JM, Johnson PWM et al, Patterns of outcome following recurrence after myeloablative therapy with autologous bone marrow transplantation for follicular lymphoma. *J Clin Oncol* 1999; **17**: 216–21.

49. Dreger P, Viehmann K, von Neuhoff N et al, Autografting of highly purified peripheral blood progenitor cells following myeloablative therapy in patients with lymphoma: a prospective study of the long-term effects on tumor eradication, reconstitution of hematopoiesis and immune recovery. *Bone Marrow Transplant* 1999; **24**: 153–61.

50. Hundsdorfer P, Fruehauf S, Haberkorn M et al, Comparison of different lymphoma cell purging modalities: An experimental study with K422 lymphoma cells. *Acta Haematol* 1999; **101**: 185–92.

51. Salles G, Moullet I, Charlot C et al, In vivo purging with rituximab before autologous peripheral blood progenitor cell transplantation in lymphoma patients. *Blood* 1999; **94**: 141a.

52. Buckstein R, Imrie K, Spaner D et al, Stem cell function and engraftment is not affected by 'in vivo purging' with rituximab for autologous stem cell treatment

for patients with low-grade non-Hodgkin's lymphoma. *Semin Oncol* 1999; **26**: 115–22.

53. Verdonck LF, Allogeneic versus autologous bone marrow transplantation for refractory and recurrent low-grade non-Hodgkin's lymphoma: updated results of the Utrecht experience. *Leuk Lymphoma* 1999; **34**: 129–36.

54. Bendandi M, Gocke CD, Kobrin CB et al, Complete molecular remissions induced by patient-specific vaccination plus granulocyte-monocyte colony-stimulating factor against lymphoma. *Nature Med* 1999; **5**: 1171–7.

55. Cotter FE, Antisense therapy of hematologic malignancies. *Semin Hematol* 1999; **36**: 9–14.

56. Kuss B, Cotter F, Antisense: time to shoot the messenger. *Ann Oncol* 1999; **10**: 495–503.

57. Warzocha K, Antisense strategy in hematological malignancies. *Cytokines Cell Mol Ther* 1999; **5**: 15–23.

5
Mantle cell lymphoma

Martin Dreyling, Tanja Meyer, Wolfgang Hiddemann

INTRODUCTION

Although this subentity of malignant lymphoma had already been described almost two decades ago as centrocytic lymphoma (in the Kiel classification) or intermediate differentiated lymphocytic lymphoma (in the Modified Working Classification), it was not until the introduction of the Revised European–American Lymphoma (REAL) and World Health Organization (WHO) classifications that mantle cell lymphoma (MCL) became generally accepted as a distinct entity. The name MCL is derived from the physiological counterpart of the lymphoma cells, which is believed to comprise cells of the mantle zone of lymph node follicles, representing a subset of naive pregerminal center cells. Accordingly, in most cases of MCL, no somatic hypermutations of the immunoglobulin (Ig) genes can be detected, in contrast to other lymphomas of germinal follicular (lymphoma) or postgerminal origin (multiple myeloma). In a few cases of MCL, somatic hypermutations are found – the biological significance of this observation is unclear.[1]

MORPHOLOGY

MCL may present with a broad cytological and histological spectrum, which complicates any diagnosis based on morphology alone.[2] Cytologically, two types of MCL have been described: the classical form and its variants (small cell, blastoid, and pleomorphic MCL).[3] In classical MCL, atypical cells appear monotonously small- to medium-sized with irregular, cleaved nuclei, moderately coarse chromatin, inconspicuous nucleoli, and scanty cytoplasm. The small cell variant is characterized by round nuclei, and may resemble chronic lymphocytic leukemia (CLL). The blastoid variant is found in 10–20% of cases. Some authors further discriminate between a pleomorphic form with larger (centroblast-like) cells with more finely dispersed chromatin and a blastic form with smaller irregular blast-like nuclei and prominent nucleoli.[4]

With regard to the tumor architecture, a diffuse and a nodular growth pattern (with or without germinal centers) may be discriminated. Nevertheless, in the largest systematical pathological review published so far, there was a large overlap of both subsets and poor reproducibility.[4]

Variant cytology and a diffuse growth pattern tend to have a worse prognosis in comparison with classical MCL and nodular architecture respectively. However, the strongest prognostic factor seems to be the proliferation rate as determined either by the number of mitoses or the Ki67 index.[5] This is especially interesting in view of the characteristic cyclin D1 overexpression in virtually all cases of MCL.

The immunohistologic features show a characteristic phenotype. Usually, the neoplastic cells coexpress the B-cell markers CD19 and CD20 as well as the pan-T-cell antigen CD5 in the absence of CD10, similarly to CLL. In contrast to CLL, MCL is usually CD23⁻. An even more specific marker may be CD79a, which is highly expressed in MCL whereas it is hardly detectable on CLL cells. In contrast to other subentities of malignant lymphomas (diffuse large cell, follicular, and lymphoplasmocytoid lymphomas), MCL and CLL cells express CD43 in more than 90% of cases. For further differentiation, additional adhesion markers may be useful.[6]

The quantitative evaluation of various cellular adhesion molecules (CD11a, CD29, CD49d, CD54, CD58) revealed significantly different expressions in low-grade lymphomas (MCL, CLL, and follicular lymphoma) and in aggressive lymphomas (with the latter having high expression levels).[7] In contrast, Angelopoulou et al[8] found a specific expression pattern in MCL, with high CD54 and low L-selectin and CD11c. Further studies are necessary to elucidate the biological significance of this observation. In addition, the monoclonal B cells of MCL almost always express surface immunoglobulin M (sIgM) and often sIgD; in about 20% of cases, sIgG is detectable as well. In approximately 60% of cases, MCL express monoclonal Ig λ light chains (reversed κ to λ light chain ratio).

BIOLOGY

The cytogenetic hallmark of MCL is the chromosomal translocation t(11;14)(q13;q32). The molecular mechanisms of this rearrangement involve an illegitimate VDJ recombinase activity during Ig heavy-chain gene rearrangement. From the pregerminal stage of MCL cells, it can be concluded that t(11;14) occurs during an early stage of VDJ recombination. In contrast, Stamatopoulos et al[9] found that the t(11;14) may occur at a more mature stage of B-cell ontogeny than was previously thought. Various recombination-targeting motifs in the MTC region suggest that the genomic alterations in MCL take place during VH-to-DJH rearrangement.

The putative oncogene *CCDN1* (formerly called *PRAD1*) deregulated by the t(11;14) is located approximately 120 kb telomeric from the major breakpoint cluster region. By juxtaposition to the constitutionally activated Ig promotor, the gene product cyclin D1 is overexpressed in virtually all cases of MCL but is only rarely detected in other hematopoietic neoplasias (atypical CLL and hairy cell leukemia). In some rare cases of multiple myeloma, the t(11;14)(q13;q32) is found as well, but, in contrast to MCL, the breakpoint cluster spreads over a wide genomic region.[10]

Cyclin D1 plays an important role in cell cycle regulation by propelling cells from the G_1 checkpoint into S phase. The activated cyclin D1/cyclin-dependent kinase (CDK) complex results in the phosphorylation and inactivation of the well-known tumor suppressor retinoblastoma protein (pRb). The transcription factor E2F is released and the cells pass into S phase by transactivation of multiple mitosis-associated genes.

Interestingly, although cyclin D1 is overexpressed in all MCL, the proliferation rate in classical MCL ranges between 5% and 40%, whereas in variant forms, a proliferative fraction of 40–70% is found.[11] However, overexpression of cyclin D1 alone is not sufficient to induce lymphoma development in transgenic mice; additional genetic alterations are necessary to promote the clinical manifestation. Accordingly, secondary alterations are a frequent event and important prognostic determinants in MCL.

In more than 80% of MCL, secondary alterations have been detected, 40–50% with complex cytogenetic alterations.[12–15] In a recent study of 45 cases of MCL (32 typical, 13 blastoid variants) by comparative genomic hybridization (CGH), the most frequent events were gains of chromosomes 3q, 7p, 8q, 9q34, 12q and 18q, and losses of chromosomes 1p, 6q, 9p, 10p14–p15, 11q14–q23, 13 and 17p. In addition, high-level DNA amplifications in 11 different regions of the genome were identified (predominantly in 3q27–q29, 18q23, and Xq28). Gains of 12q and high-level DNA amplifications of 10p12–p13 were identified as *CDK4* and *BMI-1* amplifications. The relevant target genes of chromosomal imbalances, especially gains of 3q, gains of 12q, and losses of 9p, were associated with shorter survival of the patients and had a strong prognostic significance.[16]

Similar results were reported in other studies using conventional cytogenetics and/or interphase fluorescence in situ hybridization (FISH). Analyzing 42 cases of MCL, Cuneo et al[13] found that the most frequent genetic alterations were 13q14 deletion (52.3%), 17p deletion (28.5%), and total or partial trisomy 12 (26%). Interestingly, 13q14 deletion represents an early secondary event, and is also found in other subtypes of NHL, especially CLL.[12] The significant differences between blastoid and typical MCL were gains of 3q, 7p and 12q, and losses of 17p (which correlated with *p53* gene deletions and mutations). Only trisomy 12 was associated with a shorter survival, but the increasing degree of karyotype complexity correlated best with a poor prognosis.[13]

The target genes of the 9p21 and the 17p13 alterations are the deletions of *p16INK4A* (*MTS1, CDKN2*) and *p53*, respectively. *p16* encodes an inhibitor of the cyclin D1/CDK complex. Similarly, *p53* may effect cell proliferation via upregulation of expression of the *p21* gene (another CDK inhibitor), which regulates cell cycle activity at various checkpoints. Thus, the effects of cyclin D1 overexpression at the G_1 checkpoint can be further enhanced by additional genetic alterations, which may represent the most important biological determinants of clinical outcome in MCL. In addition, mutations of the tumor suppressor genes *p53* and *p16* closely correlate with secondary transformation into highly malignant forms and the morphology of blastoid variants.

Another frequent secondary alteration in MCL is the cytogenetic deletion at 11q21–23, which has been further characterized at the molecular level. Monni et al[17] detected deletions of chromosomal band 11q21–23 in about 50% of cases (20/41) and constructed a YAC (yeast artificial chromosome) contigue, which spans several megabases and covers the commonly deleted region. Another group found the *ATM* gene as the minimal consensus deletion of 11q21–23. Additionally, Schaffner et al[18] identified *ATM* mutations in MCL with hemizygous 11q deletion, indicating that *ATM* is the relevant candidate gene of the region and may play an important role in B-cell tumorigenesis in MCL as well as CLL.

CLINICAL PRESENTATION

MCL represents 5–10% of all non-Hodgkin's lymphomas (NHL) in Europe. Patients have a median age of over 60 years, with a predominance of the male sex. The disease is mostly diagnosed at advanced Ann Arbor stages (>80% stage IV) and a large tumorous mass, a generalized lymphadenopathy, and the involvement of bone marrow, liver or other extranodal manifestation.[5] In 60% of cases, massive splenomegaly, hepatomegaly, and bulky disease is present at initial diagnosis, but B symptoms are found in less than 50%. Another frequently overseen extranodal manifestation is multiple lymphomatous polyposis (MLP), which is characterized by multiple polyps involving long segments of the gastrointestinal (GI) tract.[19] However, MLP is a heterogenous group, since cases with malignant cells derived from pregerminal as well as germinal center B cells have been described.[20]

Additionally, some patients present with elevated leukocyte counts and massive spleen enlargement, and without superficial lymphadenopathy.[21] These patients have a significantly worse outcome in comparison with the overall group of MCL.[2]

Especially in relapsed MCL, the disease may present with atypical features. In a retrospective analysis of four patients with CNS involvement, malignant cells could be detected in the spinal fluid in all cases, whereas parenchymal brain infiltrations were found in two cases. Although treated with intrathecal chemotherapy, survival after CNS lymphoma was a maximum of 55 days without any response to therapy.[22]

NEW DIAGNOSTIC FEATURES

In 60% of cases of MCL, bone marrow involvement can be detected with histo-logical and immunohistochemical analyses; however, the use of additional detection methods may result in an even higher infiltration rate. In cases diag-nosed as inconclusive, amplification of the Ig heavy-chain (IgH) complemen-tarity-determining region (CDR3) by PCR can be helpful.[23] Bertoni et al[24] examined blood samples from 16 patients with pathologically reviewed MCL by PCR. In 44%, t(11;14)(q13;q32) were found, a further 44% showed the presence of circulating neoplastic B cells (amplification of monoclonal CDR3 and Ig κ light-chain rearrangements). Only in 12% could PCR not detect circu-lating lymphoma cells, indicating that PCR is diagnostically important.[24] In another recent study, the highest sensitivity was achieved by interphase FISH with *CCND1* and *IgH* probes encompassing the breakpoint regions of the t(11;14)(q13;q32). In all 51 cases of patients with MCL analyzed, FISH deter-mined a specific fusion signal, in comparison with 50% detected by PCR and 70% by conventional cytogenetic analysis. Moreover, this technique is widely applicable.[25]

As mentioned earlier, the diagnosis of MCL may be difficult when based on morphology alone. In particular, cytological analysis of bone marrow samples only may lead to misinterpretation, because of an altered morphology com-pared with lymph node histology. Therefore additional immunophenotyping with BCL2, CD5, CD10, CD23 and CD43, or molecular analysis (PCR of *IgH* rearrangement), may lead to an accurate estimation of bone marrow involve-ment.[23,26]

Similarly, diagnosis of mantle cell leukemia (the leukemic phase of MCL) may be improved by immunophenotyping and cytomorphology of the periph-eral blood.[27]

In fact, it had been suggested that in all atypical CLL cases, cyclin D1 overex-pression should be systemically determined. In a retrospective study of 192 cases of chronic lymphoproliferative disorders (CLD), Levy et al[21] identified 40 cases, 10 of which were cyclin D1-positive and showed a uniform clinical presentation with leukocytosis, massive spleen enlargement, and no superficial lymph-adenopathy. Compared with the cyclin D1-negative cases, the outcome was very poor, with a median survival of 10 month only. Thus Levy et al[21] proposed that unclassified CLD should be reclassified as mantle cell leukemia, because of the characteristic cyclin D1 overexpression and the typical clinical outcome.

THERAPY

With conventional treatment, the clinical outcome of MCL is disastrous, with a median survival of three years and virtually no long-term survival. New drugs such as single-agent fludarabine phosphate have only a moderate activity, with remission rates of 40%.[28]

Immunotherapy with anti-CD20 antibody also has only a limited efficacy in MCL. In comparison with previous series, Nguyen et al[29] found a significantly lower overall remission rate of only 20% of cases (2/10 partial remissions).

Another biological modifier that may have a benefit in MCL is interferon-α (IFN-α) in induction or maintenance therapy. However, the series published so far have shown only a tendency in favor of IFN-α, mostly because of the small number of cases analyzed.

A promising option is high-dose radiochemotherapy with subsequent stem cell retransfusion. However, although previous series suggested a superior outcome, this therapeutic option is hampered by severe late toxicity, including secondary leukemia or other long-term side-effects. Re et al[30] reported a case of progressive multifocal leukencephalopathy as another example of late toxicity.

Additionally, some authors claim that survival curves after autologous stem cell transplantation do not reach a plateau. This may be a result of contamination of the harvested blood stem cells with circulating MCL cells. In fact, previous attempts purging peripheral blood stem cells (PBSC) did not achieve a PCR conversion. An innovative approach may be the ex vivo purging of PBSC with chemotherapy.[31]

The only curative approach so far is allogeneic bone marrow transplantation, which is hampered by high early and late mortality mostly due to infectious complications. A new approach may be the application of non-myeloablative regimens (minitransplant), which is based on the immunological graft-versus-lymphoma effect. In fact, Grigg et al[32] described one patient with chemorefractory MCL, who achieved HLA-identical stem cells after non-myeloablative chemotherapy and progressed early post transplant. With the onset of severe graft-versus-host disease (GvHD) following cessation of cyclosporin A, the patient entered remission, suggesting a powerful graft-versus-lymphoma effect.

Khouri et al[33] confirmed the efficacy of allogeneic hematopoietic transplantation in 16 cases of advanced-stage MCL. After cytoreductive therapy (HYPER-CVAD) and consecutive hematopoietic transplantation, 9 of 16 patients remained alive and progression-free after a median follow-up time of 24 months. Moreover, molecular remission was achieved in 5 of 7 patients analyzed. These data strongly support the role of the graft-versus-lymphoma effect in MCL.

Alternatively, molecular defined approaches with selective CDK inhibition (flavopiridol) may be worthwhile, although the clinical effect of monotherapy reported so far is limited.

REFERENCES

1. Peng HZ, Du MQ, Koulis A et al, Nonimmunoglobulin gene hypermutation in germinal center B cells. *Blood* 1999; **93**: 2167–72.

2. Wong KF, Chan JK, So CC et al, Mantle cell lymphoma in leukemic phase: characterization of its broad cytologic spectrum with emphasis on the importance of distinction from other chronic lymphoproliferative disorders. *Cancer* 1999; **86**: 850–7.

3. Campo E, Raffeld M, Jaffee ES, Mantle-cell lymphoma. *Semin Hematol* 1999; **36**: 115–27.

4. Tiemann M, Schrader C, Dreyling MH et al, for the European MCL Study Group, Pathology, proliferation indices and survival in 304 patients. *Ann Oncol* 1999; **10**: 29.

5. Dreyling MH, Hiddemann W, for the European MCL Study Group, Prognostic factors in mantle cell lymphoma: clinical characteristics, pathology and cell proliferation. *Proc Am Soc Clin Oncol* 1999; **18**: 3a.

6. Lai R, Weiss LM, Chang KL et al, Frequency of CD43 expression in non-Hodgkin lymphoma. A survey of 742 cases and further characterization of rare CD43+ follicular lymphomas. *Am J Clin Pathol* 1999; **111**: 488–94.

7. Jacob MC, Agrawal S, Chaperot L et al, Quantification of cellular adhesion molecules on malignant B cells from non-Hodgkin's lymphoma. *Leukemia* 1999; **13**: 1428–33.

8. Angelopoulou MK, Kontopidou FN, Pangalis GA, Adhesion molecules in B-chronic lymphoproliferative disorders. *Semin Hematol* 1999; **36**: 178–97.

9. Stamatopoulos K, Kosmas C, Belessi C et al, Molecular analysis of bcl-1/IgH junctional sequences in mantle cell lymphoma: potential mechanism of the t(11;14) chromosomal translocation. *Br J Haematol* 1999; **105**: 190–7.

10. Ronchetti D, Finelli P, Richelda R et al, Molecular analysis of 11q13 break-points in multiple myeloma. *Blood* 1999; **93**: 1330–7.

11. Fiel-Gan MD Almeida LM, Rose DC et al, Proliferative fraction, bcl-1 gene translocation, and p53 mutation status as markers in mantle cell lymphoma. *Int J Mol Med* 1999; **3**: 373–9.

12. Cuneo A, Bigoni R, Rigolin GM et al, 13q14 deletion in non-Hodgkin's lymphoma: correlation with clinicopathologic features. *Haematologica* 1999; **84**: 589–93.

13. Cuneo A, Bigoni R, Rigolin GM et al, Cytogenetic profile of lymphoma of follicle mantle lineage: correlation with clinicobiologic features. *Blood* 1999; **93**: 1372–80.

14. Espinet B, Solé F, Woessner S et al, Translocation (11;14)(q13;q32) and preferential involvement of chromosomes 1, 2, 9, 13, and 17 in mantle cell lymphoma. *Cancer Genet Cytogenet* 1999; **111**: 92–8.

15. Wlodarska I, Pittaluga S, Hagemeijer A et al, Secondary chromosome changes in mantle cell lymphoma. *Haematologica* 1999; **84**: 594–9.

16. Beà S, Ribas M, Hernandez JM et al, Increased number of chromosomal imbalances and high-level DNA amplifications in mantle cell lymphoma are associated with blastoid variants. *Blood* 1999; **93**: 4365–74.

17. Monni O, Zhu Y, Franssila K et al, Molecular characterization of deletion at 11q22.1–23.3 in mantle cell lymphoma. *Br J Haematol* 1999; **104**: 665–71.

18. Schaffner C, Stilgenbauer S, Rappold GA et al, Somatic ATM mutations indicate a pathogenic role of ATM in B-cell chronic lymphocytic leukemia. *Blood* 1999; **94**: 748–53.

19. Isaacson PG, Gastrointestinal lymphomas of T- and B-cell types. *Mod Pathol* 1999; **12**: 151–8.

20. Hashimoto Y, Nakamura N, Kuze T et al, Multiple lymphomatous polyposis of the gastrointestinal tract is a hetero-

genous group that includes mantle cell lymphoma and follicular lymphoma: analysis of somatic mutation of immunoglobulin heavy chain gene variable region. *Hum Pathol* 1999; **30**: 581–7.

21. Levy V, Ugo V, Delmer A et al, Cyclin D1 overexpression allows identification of an aggressive subset of leukemic lymphoproliferative disorder. *Leukemia* 1999; **13**: 1343–51.

22. Oinonen R, Franssila K, Elonen E, Central nervous system involvement in patients with mantle cell lymphoma. *Ann Hematol* 1999; **78**: 145–9.

23. Pittaluga S, Tierens A, Dodoo YL et al, How reliable is histologic examination of bone marrow trephine biopsy specimens for the staging of non-Hodgkin lymphoma? A study of hairy cell leukemia and mantle cell lymphoma involvement of the bone marrow trephine specimen by histologic, immunohistochemical, and polymerase chain reaction techniques. *Am J Clin Pathol* 1999; **111**: 179–84.

24. Bertoni F, Roggero E, Luscieti P et al, Clonality assessment in blood of patients with mantle cell lymphoma. *Leuk Lymphoma* 1999; **32**: 375–9.

25. Li JY, Gaillard F, Moreau A et al, Detection of translocation t(11;14)(q13;q32) in mantle cell lymphoma by fluorescence in situ hybridization. *Am J Pathol* 1999; **154**: 1449–52.

26. Rassidakis GZ, Tani E, Svedmur E et al, Diagnosis and subclassification of follicle center and mantle cell lymphomas on fine-needle aspirates: a cytologic and immunocytochemical approach based on the Revised European–American Lymphoma (REAL) classification. *Cancer* 1999; **87**: 216–23.

27. Dunphy CH, Hancock JC, Rodriguez JJ et al, Blastic mantle cell leukemia: a previously undescribed form. *J Clin Lab Anal* 1999; **13**: 112–15.

28. Foran JM, Rohatiner AZ, Coiffier B et al, Multicenter phase II study of fludarabine phosphate for patients with newly diagnosed lymphoplasmacytoid lymphoma, Waldenström's macroglobulinemia, and mantle-cell lymphoma. *J Clin Oncol* 1999; **17**: 546–53.

29. Nguyen DT, Amess JA, Doughty H et al, IDEC-C2B8 anti-CD20 (rituximab) immunotherapy in patients with low-grade non-Hodgkin's lymphoma and lymphoproliferative disorders: evaluation of response on 48 patients. *Eur J Haematol* 1999; **62**: 76–82.

30. Re D, Bamborschke S, Feiden W et al, Progressive multifocal leukoencephalopathy after autologous bone marrow transplantation and alpha-interferon immunotherapy. *Bone Marrow Transplant* 1999; **23**: 295–8.

31. Lemoli RM, Visani G, Leopardi K et al, Autologous transplantation of chemotherapy-purged PBSC collections from high-risk leukemia patients: a pilot study. *Bone Marrow Transplant* 1999; **23**: 235–41.

32. Grigg A, Bardy P, Byron K et al, Fludarabine-based non-myeloablative chemotherapy followed by infusion of HLA-identical stem cells for relapsed leukaemia and lymphoma. *Bone Marrow Transplant* 1999; **23**: 107–10.

33. Khouri F, Lee M-S, Romaguera J et al, Allogenetic hematopoietic transplantation for mantle-cell lymphoma: molecular remission and evidence of graft-versus-malignancy. *Ann Oncol* 1999; **10**: 1293–9.

6
Diffuse large cell lymphomas

John E Godwin, Richard I Fisher

STATE OF THE ART: OVERVIEW OF DIFFUSE LARGE CELL LYMPHOMAS

Non-Hodgkin's lymphomas (NHLs) are expected to produce 55 000 new cases in the USA in the year 2000, making this the fifth most common cancer in men and women.[1] NHLs are heterogeneous lymphoproliferative malignancies, with different clinical behaviors and underlying biology. Historically, NHLs were classified principally by morphologic features, primarily the presence or absence of a follicular (nodular pattern), and the size and shape of the malignant cells. However, with six major classification schemes in place, there was difficulty in understanding which treatments were effective. In 1982, the results of a consensus classification were published as the Working Formulation (WF) (Table 6.1), which served as a uniform translation between existing classification schemes and divided all NHLs into three prognostic grades – low, intermediate, or high – based on the similarity of the survival curves of patients after therapy.[2] Many clinical investigators, especially in the USA, subsequently found it more convenient to divide NHLs into two categories – indolent and aggressive. In this frame of reference, the indolent NHLs were WF categories A–E, and the remaining categories F–J were considered aggressive. Although the WF was easy to understand and use by the clinician, an ever-accumulating body of evidence indicated that many distinct diseases were being grouped together in this classification scheme. In 1994, the International Lymphoma Study Group proposed the Revised European American Lymphoma (REAL) classification encompassing all lymphoproliferative neoplasms[3] (Table 6.2). This proposal defined 'real' disease entities, based on clinical and pathologic uniformity. The clinical significance and reproducibility of the proposed classification was confirmed in an international population-based study.[4] The newest classification scheme is from the World Health Organization (WHO); this proposal maintains the basic organization of the REAL classification with minor modifications, and updates tentative categories from that classification.[5] Using the REAL classification, the entity we review here is termed diffuse large B-cell lymphoma (DLBCL) – or commonly diffuse large cell lymphoma (DLCL).

Table 6.1 The Working Formulation

Grade	International Working Formulation
Low grade	A. Small lymphocytic (SL), consistent with chronic lymphocytic leukemia B. Follicular (FSC), predominantly small cleaved cell, diffuse areas C. Follicular mixed (FM), small cleaved cell and large cell
Intermediate grade	D. Follicular (FL), predominantly large cell E. Diffuse, small cleaved cell (DSC) F. Diffuse, mixed (DM), small cleaved cell and large cell G. Diffuse, large cell (DL), cleaved cell or noncleaved cell
High grade	H. Immunoblastic, large cell (IBL) I. Lymphoblastic (LL), convoluted cell or nonconvoluted cell J. Small noncleaved cell (SNC), Burkitt's or non-Burkitt's

Treatment for non-localized DLCL with the so-called 'first-generation' regimen, CHOP (cyclophosphamide, doxorubicin, vincristine, and prednisone) has been studied extensively in national cooperative-group trials, and CHOP has emerged as the current standard therapy. This verdict was conclusively demonstrated in the Southwest Oncology Group (SWOG) Trial 8516, conducted in collaboration with the Eastern Cooperative Oncology Group (ECOG), comparing standard therapy (CHOP) with the 'second-' and 'third-generation' chemotherapy regimens* m-BACOD, ProMACE–CytaBOM, or MACOP-B in patients with stage II–IV disease, and WF intermediate-grade or high-grade lymphomas (D–H, and J, excluding lymphoblastic lymphoma).[6] After over six years, there is still no difference between CHOP and the third-generation regimens in terms of progression-free survival rate, with five-year estimates varying from 33% to 38%, or in overall survival rate, with five-year estimates varying from 45% to 46%. This result surprised those who had observed phase II trials of the third-generation regimens demonstrate increased complete remission rates and survival rates of 55–65%. How could such disparate results occur in the single-institution phase II studies and the subsequent national phase II as well as the final national phase III trials? One key explanation emerging is that DLCL, as identified in any of the current

---

* m-BACOD is methotrexate (with leucovorin rescue), bleomycin, doxorubicin, cyclophosphamide, vincristine, and dexamethasone; ProMACE–CytaBOM is prednisone, doxorubicin, cyclophosphamide, and etoposide, followed by cytarabine, bleomycin, vincristine, and methotrexate (with leucovorin rescue); MACOP-B is methotrexate (with leucovorin rescue), doxorubicin, cyclophosphamide, vincristine, bleomycin, prednisone, and trimethoprim–sulfamethoxazole.

Table 6.2 REAL classification

B-cell neoplasms	T-cell and putative NK-cell neoplasms
I. Precursor B-cell neoplasm Precursor B-lymphoblastic leukemia/lymphoma	*I. Precursor T-cell neoplasm* Precursor T-lymphoblastic lymphoma/leukemia
II. Peripheral B-cell neoplasms	*II. Peripheral T-cell and NK-cell neoplasms*
A. B-cell chronic lymphocytic leukemia (CLL)/prolymphocytic leukemia (PLL)/small lymphocytic	A. T-cell chronic lymphocytic leukemia (CLL)/prolymphocytic leukemia (PLL)
B. Lymphoplasmacytoid lymphoma/immunocytoma	B. Large granular lymphocyte leukemia 1. T-cell type 2. NK-cell type
C. Mantle cell lymphoma	C. Mycosis fungoides/Sézary syndrome
D. Follicle center cell lymphoma, follicular 1. Provisional cytologic grades: I (small cell), II (mixed small and large cell), III (large cell) 2. Provisional subtype: diffuse, predominantly small cell type	D. Peripheral T-cell lymphomas, unspecified 1. Provisional cytologic categories: medium sized cell, mixed medium and large cell, large cell, lymphoepitheloid cell 2. Provisional subtype: hepatosplenic γ/δ T-cell lymphoma 3. Provisional subtype: subcutaneous panniculitic T-cell lymphoma
E. Marginal zone B-cell lymphoma 1. Extranodal (MALT-type $\pm$ monocytoid B cells) 2. Provisional subtype: nodal ($\pm$ monocytoid B cells)	
F. Provisional entity: splenic marginal zone lymphoma ($\pm$ villous lymphocytes)	E. Angioimmunoblastic T-cell lymphoma
G. Hairy cell leukemia	F. Angiocentric lymphoma
H. Plasmacytoma/plasma cell myeloma	G. Intestinal T-cell lymphoma ($\pm$ enteropathy)
I. Diffuse large B-cell lymphoma Subtype: primary mediastinal (thymic) B-cell lymphoma	H. Adult T-cell lymphoma/leukemia
J. Burkitt's lymphoma	I. Anaplastic large cell lymphoma 1. CD30$^+$ cell type 2. T-cell type 3. Null-cell types
K. Provisional entity: high-grade B-cell lymphoma, Burkitt-like	J. Provisional entity: anaplastic large cell lymphoma, Hodgkin-like

$\pm$, with or without.

classification schemes, is not a uniform disease. Data supporting this concept are clear from recent studies on prognostic indexes. The International Non-Hodgkin's Lymphoma Prognostic Factors Index (IPI) utilized pretreatment prognostic factors in a sample of over 5000 patients with lymphomas to develop a predictive model of outcome for aggressive NHL.[7] The majority of patients had received doxorubicin-based chemotherapy regimens. In an analysis of 2031 aggressive lymphoma patients (WF categories F, G, and H) of all ages, five pretreatment characteristics were found to be independent significant predictors of death: age (60 years or less versus over 60), tumor stage (I or II (localized) versus III or IV (advanced)), the number of extra nodal sites of involvement (none or one versus more than one), patient ECOG performance status (0 or 1 (ambulatory) versus ≥ 2 (not ambulatory); equivalent Karnofsky scores ≥ 80 versus ≤ 70), and serum lactate dehydrogenase (LDH) level (≤ 1 times normal versus >1 times normal). Each of the individual factors had comparable relative risks, and thus could be summed together. The resulting model identified four risk groups with predicted five-year survival rates: low risk (0–1) 73%, low intermediate risk (2) 51%, high intermediate risk (3) 43%, and high risk (4–5) 26%. The increased risk of death was due to both a lower complete response (CR) rate and a higher rate of relapse from CR. For example, patients in the high-risk IPI group had a CR rate of 44% and a five-year survival rate of only 26%, as compared with a CR rate of 87% and a five-year survival rate of 73% in patients in the low-risk IPI group. The IPI has provided us with a methodology to compare the patients entering various clinical trials, and explained the variation in treatment outcomes initially attributed to the effect of 'third-generation' chemotherapy. The percentage of patients with favorable (low) IPI scores in the original National Cancer Institute trial of Pro-MACE–CytaBOM (44%) was almost twice that in the subsequent SWOG-8516 phase III study (22%).[6,8] The differences in outcome caused by these imbalances in patient prognostic factors can easily exceed any treatment differences between the actual therapies. It is important to remember that these clinical factors are proxy measures for the underlying biologic and molecular variation within the large cell lymphoma disease category.

Our understanding of the biology of diffuse large B-cell lymphomas is still in its infancy. Each of the categories of B-cell malignancy has been traced to a particular stage in normal B-cell development. It is axiomatic that a component of the biology of a malignant cell is inherited from its normal cellular ancestors. Virtually all Non-Hodgkin's B-cell lymphomas are derived from B-lineage cells that have completed both immunoglobulin heavy-chain and light-chain (IgH and IgL) recombination and can express functional Ig protein. Additionally NHL can be divided into pre-germinal center (pre-GC), germinal center (GC), and post-germinal center (post-GC) categories. The rearranged immunoglobulin genes in DLCL bear mutations characteristic of somatic hypermutation, an antibody-diversification process that normally occurs within the GC of lymph nodes.[9] Evidence suggests that DLCL arises from B cells from within the GC or at a later stage of differentiation (post-GC). Three recurring karyotypic abnormalities have been recognized in DLCLs: t(14;18) with *BLC2* overexpression in approximately 30%; 3q27 rearrangements with *BCL6* overexpression in 30–40%; and t(8;14) with c-*MYC* overexpression in some cases. The proximity of these oncogenes to the immunoglobulin gene caused by the translocation results in deregulation and increased expression of the gene product. Clues to *BCL2* gene function came from transfection constructs and transgenic mice.[10,11] Cells taken from *BCL2*-transgenic mice were found to survive long periods of time in culture without cell division, and thus BCL2 protein was found to prevent programmed cell death (apoptosis). BCL2 belongs to a family of proteins, now estimated at over 15 different members, regulating programmed cell death. Some BCL2 family members, such as BCLX$_L$, have anti-apoptotic roles, while others, such as BAX, are pro-apoptotic. These proteins can somehow register diverse forms of intracellular damage and integrate these signals to decide an apoptotic outcome, by a mechanism that is incompletely understood. Approximately 35% of DLCLs demonstrate translocation of chromosome 3 band q27, the target of which has been termed *BCL6*.[12] The product of the *BCL6* gene is a zinc-finger DNA-binding protein.[13] However, rather than being a transcription activator like c-MYC, BCL6 represses transcription of target genes, which are yet to be elucidated.[14] Translocations of 3q27 involve a variety of chromosome partners, including Ig loci on chromosomes 14, 2, and 22. In normal B cells, BCL6 protein is only found in germinal centers, and in fact it may be required for GC formation, since no GCs form in *BCL6*-knockout mice.[15] The chromosomal translocation t(8;14) is characteristic of Burkitt's lymphoma, and is associated with the overexpression of c-*MYC* a member of the helix–loop–helix family of DNA-binding transcription factors. DLCLs rarely have t(8;14) detected. Overexpression of c-*MYC* activates transcription and promotes cell division, though paradoxically overexpression can induce apoptosis unless other mutations are present to inhibit apoptosis, such as BCL2 expression.[16] Several studies have indicated that some of these molecular factors, such as increased expression of BCL2, are independent prognostic markers in DLCLs in addition to the use of the IPI.[17,18] Mutations of *p53* occur commonly in solid tumors, but appear uncommon in lymphomas. Alterations in *p53* are more common in aggressive lymphomas, and are associated with poor prognosis.[19,20]

This chapter will summarize literature on the developments in the pathology, biology, and treatment of DLCLs in the past year. Based on the facts that fewer than 50% of all patients are cured and that we can now identify subsets of patients with even lower cure rates, it is absolutely essential that oncologists develop new and improved therapeutic approaches for patients with advanced-stage, aggressive-histology NHL.

LITERATURE REVIEW: PATHOLOGY/BIOLOGY OF DIFFUSE LARGE CELL LYMPHOMAS

The REAL classification of NHL and lymphoproliferative disorders has been tentatively updated in the new WHO classification proposal, under development since 1995 by the European Association of Pathologists (EAHP) and the Society for Hematopathology (SH).[5] The WHO classification is more ambitious than the REAL classification, and proposes to classify all hematological malignancies, including lymphoid, myeloid, histiocytic, and mast cell neoplasms. The WHO approach to classification is based on the principle adopted in the REAL scheme, that a classification is a tabulation of 'real' disease entities, which are established by their morphology, immunophenotype, genetic features, and clinical features. A Clinical Advisory Committee (CAC) of international hematologists and oncologists was formed for the WHO organizers, to ensure that the classification will be suitable to clinicians. One somewhat controversial conclusion of the CAC is that clinical grouping of lymphoid neoplasms is neither necessary nor desirable. This would eliminate the common clinical designations of aggressive and indolent lymphoma. The recommendation of the CAC is that patient treatment be determined by the specific type of lymphoma, with supplementation of tumor grade, if applicable, and prognostic factors such as the IPI.[21] There is still controversy regarding some of the proposed lymphoma designations in the REAL and WHO schemes. The disorder 'primary mediastinal (thymic) B-cell lymphoma' (PMLBL), classified as a subtype of large cell lymphoma in the REAL classification, may at times present unusual morphological appearance and be difficult to distinguish. The disorder is believed to arise from a native B-cell population of the thymus, thus representing a primary extranodal large-B-cell lymphoma of the thymus.[22] A study from the University of Nebraska compared 43 cases of mediastinal large-cell lymphomas with 352 control, non-mediastinal lymphomas.[23] In this study, there was no difference in CR rate, disease-free survival or overall survival between cases of PMLBL and control lymphomas, and a younger median age in PMLBL was the only clinical feature that was significantly different. Although the earlier age of onset, slight female predominance, mediastinal location, and size of the mass may justify the recognition of primary large cell lymphomas as a clinical syndrome, these authors do not favor the addition of a distinct category, or clinical entity, for PMLBL. Another classification question in the REAL scheme concerns DLCL subtyping. No subtypes of DLCL are recognized in REAL, in contrast to the Working Formulation, because subclassifications were considered to lack both reproducibility and clinical significance. Others, however, claim that patients with immunoblastic lymphoma have a worse prognosis than patients with other types of DLCL. In their retrospective review, Baars and colleagues[24] from the University of Amsterdam describe 177 patients treated in the Netherlands between 1984 and 1994 with immunoblastic (IB), centroblastic polymorphic subtype (CB-Poly), or centroblastic (CB) lymphoma as determined by a central lymphoma review panel. Patients were assigned IPI risk factors. A multivariate analysis showed that histological sub-typing was of prognostic significance, independent of the IPI. Patients with IB or CB-Poly subtype lymphoma showed significantly worse prognosis than patients with CB NHL, with a five-year disease-free survival rate of 53% for patients with CB, 32% for patients with CB-Poly, and 27% for patients with IB NHL. The authors suggest further study of this observation in prospective trials. However, it remains to be seen whether other institutions could agree with the classification scheme used by the authors, or reproduce these results. Nonetheless, the concept that the category of DLCLs contains multiple disease entities is supported by the findings using the IPI. Investigators at the Mayo Clinic have reported a study testing the hypothesis that the survival differences between the groups defined by established prognostic factors such as the IPI were due to the proliferative index of the tumor.[25] In this study, the bromo-deoxyuridine labeling index (LI), a measure of the S-phase fraction and lymphoma cell proliferation, was determined on 80 fresh initial lymphoma tumor specimens. The LI was not a significant prognostic factor for response, disease-free survival, or overall survival. Further, the LI did not explain the variation in outcome between groups defined by the IPI.

Regarding the molecular biology of lymphoma, a review by Korsmeyer[26] has updated the pro- and anti-apoptotic *BCL2* family, which are key in lymphoma pathogenesis, and expanded on newly identified members of this family, such as *BID* and *BAD*. From Tokyo, investigators have reported a study of microsatellite instability (MSI) in lymphoma and leukemia cell lines.[27] Microsatellite instability represents a defect in the DNA mismatch-repair system, and has been shown to play a role in the onset and/or progression of several human malignancies. These investigators found that 5 out of 24 (21%) of the lymphoid leukemia and lymphoma cell lines were MSI-positive. None of the myeloid leukemia cell lines were positive. These authors conclude that MSI contributes to the development of lymphoid but not to that of myeloid malignancies; these findings remain to be confirmed in additional studies.

A study reported by Rizzo et al[28] from Loyola, Chicago looked at simian virus 40 (SV40) etiologic associations in lymphoma. SV40 is causally associated with several cancers in hamsters, including mesotheliomas, osteosarcomas, ependymomas, choroid plexus tumors, and lymphomas. In humans, SV40 viral sequences have been detected most frequently in mesotheliomas, but also have been found in osteosarcomas, ependymomas, and choroid plexus tumors. Using the polymerase chain reaction (PCR), investigators tested 29 NHLs (intermediate- and high-grade), 25 post-transplant lymphoproliferative disorders, and 5 AIDS lymphomas for SV40 DNA. A very sensitive PCR analysis for SV40 sequences corresponding to the retinoblastoma (RB)-pocket binding domain SV40 tumor antigen (Tag) revealed that 10% of lymphomas, 24% of post-transplant lymphoproliferative disorders, and 2 of 5 AIDS lymphomas contained SV40 sequences. However, positive samples were then assayed for the critical SV40 regulatory region, and none of the lymphomas, only one post-transplant lymphoproliferative disorder, and one AIDS lymphoma contained these sequences. In matching experiments, 66% of mesotheliomas tested positive for SV40 for both the RB-pocket binding domain of Tag and the SV40 regulatory region. The investigators conclude that SV40 is present in most mesotheliomas in the USA, but the prevalence of SV40 is low in human lymphomas.

LITERATURE REVIEW: TREATMENT OF DIFFUSE LARGE CELL LYMPHOMAS

One significant area of progress in the last year is a proposal for the standardization of criteria for assessing response to treatment in lymphoma. Standardized guidelines for response assessment are needed to ensure comparability among clinical trials in NHL; this is particularly important in phase II trials, where the response activity of a new agent may be the only measure of effect. A simple example is that there is no general agreement on what is a 'normal size' lymph node after treatment. To achieve an international consensus, representatives from the NCI, cooperative groups, US, European and Canadian experts, and the pharmaceutical industry met to propose guidelines for response assessment.[29] The authors hope that these published guidelines will be adopted by cooperative groups and serve to improve communication among investigators and comparability among clinical trials. The consensus of the group is that normal lymph node size after treatment is 1.5 cm in the longest transverse diameter as assessed by computer-assisted tomography.

Our review of the treatment of DLCL is divided into categories based on the different approaches that are being developed:

- the identification of new active drugs for the treatment of lymphoma;
- the use of colony-stimulating factors to allow dose escalation of active but myelotoxic drugs;
- the use of strategies that may overcome the problem of resistance to chemotherapy;
- the use of monoclonal antibodies and combination of monoclonal antibodies with chemotherapy;
- ablative chemotherapy with autologous stem cell support.

Each of these approaches is discussed below.

New agents

The discovery of new drugs for the treatment of DLCL remains a difficult task for several reasons. The large number of active agents already in use, and the high number of complete remissions seen in untreated patients, means that a drug must have outstanding single-agent activity in phase II testing before it is considered for evaluation as a front line agent. Drugs that would be considered quite exciting in some solid tumors are discarded as marginally active in the lymphomas. Generally, complete remission rates in excess of 25% in phase II trials are required. In addition, many patients who are not cured by initial therapy are now considered for high-dose salvage therapy at first relapse. Thus the pool of patients available for phase II testing now consists of patients ineligible for high-dose therapy or those relapsing after that treatment.

Some agents now under investigation will be discussed. Among others, the NCI is sponsoring phase II trials of 9-aminocamptothecin, irinotecan, and arsenic trioxide. 9-Aminocamptothecin (9-AC) is a new topoisomerase I (topo I)-targeting agent. In a preliminary report, 9-AC demonstrated an overall response rate of 10/40 (25%) in heavily pretreated relapsed and refractory lymphoma patients, with chemotherapy-sensitive patients showing a 32% response rate.[30] Irinotecan (CPT-11) has a broad range of antitumor activity[31] and reports of its activity in lymphoma are found in small case series,[32] but this has encouraged a phase II evaluation sponsored by the NCI. Arsenic trioxide (As_2O_3) is an active agent in patients with acute promyelocytic leukemia, and can induce clinical remissions via induction of differentiation and programmed cell death. In vitro studies indicate substantial growth inhibition and apoptosis without differentiation, in fresh lymphoma tumor cell lines after exposure to clinical levels of arsenic trioxide.[33] A novel agent, PS-341, a proteasome inhibitor, is in phase I trial for lymphomas and refractory tumors. The ubiquitin–proteasome pathway plays a critical role in the regulated degradation of proteins involved in cell cycle control and tumor growth, and interruption of this pathway by agents such as PS-341 cause cells to undergo apoptosis.[34] Although clinical trials are continuing in many centers, at the moment there are no drugs demonstrating unequivocally high levels of single-agent activity in the DLCLs.

Colony-stimulating factors for dose escalation

Colony-stimulating factors have allowed several groups to double the dose intensity of marrow-toxic drugs such as cyclophosphamide and doxorubicin. In a cooperative group setting, SWOG has completed a randomized phase II study of dose-intensified CHOP and dose-intensified ProMACE–CytaBOM with granulocyte colony-stimulating factor (G-CSF) support. ECOG has reported a successful phase I dose-escalation study of ProMACE–CytaBOM, and has subsequently completed a phase II study of that regimen. Longer-term follow-up is required before the results of these studies can be evaluated. In addition, Shipp et al[35] reported encouraging pilot data using G-CSF to dose-escalate cyclophosphamide to 4 g/m² and doxorubicin to 70 mg/m² in a CHOP-like regimen. Subsequent phase II testing of this regimen in the Cancer and Acute Leukemia Group B (CALGB) is still being definitively analyzed, but has not confirmed the promising early results. Currently, the NCI is sponsoring phase II studies of a long-acting G-CSF, filgrastim-SD, in comparison with G-CSF in a DHAP (dexamethasone, high-dose cytarabine, and cisplatin) regimen for relapsed lymphoma, and this drug could be substituted for G-CSF in future studies of dose escalation.

Reversing drug resistance

Since pleiotropic drug resistance develops after treatment and relapse in a significant number of these patients, SWOG has conducted phase II studies with infusional CHOP plus verapamil and quinine aimed at preventing the emergence of this resistance factor. To date, we have demonstrated increased bone marrow toxicity, but have not yet seen improvement in relapse-free survival compared with historical controls treated with CHOP. Quinine and verapamil are first-generation multidrug-resistance inhibitors, and newer, more potent inhibitors of drug resistance such as PSC-388 and similar agents are currently in early clinical trials.

Treatment with monoclonal antibodies

In one of the most intensively investigated areas in lymphoma, combinations of monoclonal antibodies and chemotherapy are now being explored for DLCL. While most of the initial studies with monoclonal antibodies focused on the indolent lymphomas, Coiffier et al[36] have reported an overall response rate of 37% in relapsing or refractory aggressive lymphoma patients treated with rituximab (a chimeric anti-CD20 monoclonal antibody) alone. Similar results with rituximab alone (1 complete and 2 partial responses among 12 DLCL patients) were reported in abstract form at the 1999 American Society of Hematology by Winkler and colleagues.[37] Though responses with rituximab alone are seen in relapsed DLCL, complete responses are rare. Rituximab has been combined with CHOP chemotherapy in the treatment of newly diagnosed indolent lymphomas with few added toxicities, and with the intriguing finding of molecular remissions as defined by clearance of BCL2 by PCR.[38] Vose and colleagues[39] have recently reported in abstract form a phase II study of rituximab plus CHOP in untreated DLCL. In this study, the overall response rate was impressive, 97% (32/33), with 20 complete and 12 partial responses, and was potentially better than expected for CHOP alone. Furthermore, molecular remissions were seen, since Vose et al found 23 patients with either a unique Ig gene rearrangement or BCL2, and 11 of these (48%) had molecular remission by PCR. A phase III study is in progress at present. Rituximab is now being combined with nearly every chemotherapeutic regimen used in indolent or aggressive lymphoma, but the design of these trials is most often empiric rather than based on a biologic rationale. In addition, multiple schedules are emerging for combining the monoclonal antibody with CHOP, and this will present problems for comparing treatment results in the future.

Myeloablative chemotherapy with autologous support

Rationale for testing high-dose therapy with stem cell support in previously untreated patients with aggressive NHL was initially provided by the results of the Parma trial.[40] Patients, who had relapsed after an initial complete remission and were still under the age of 60 years with no evidence of central nervous system disease or bone marrow involvement, were first treated with two courses of conventional DHAP salvage chemotherapy. Those patients with a complete or partial response were then considered to be chemosensitive and were randomized to involved-field radiotherapy and high-dose BEAC (carmustine, etoposide, cytarabine, cyclophosphamide, and mesna) chemotherapy versus DHAP chemotherapy for four cycles followed by involved-field radiotherapy. The event-free survival rate of patients randomized to high-dose therapy was 46%, compared with 12% for patients continuing to receive salvage chemotherapy ($p = 0.001$), and overall survival was also superior in the high-dose therapy group ($p = 0.038$). This study defined high-dose therapy with stem cell support as the treatment of choice for relapsed aggressive lymphomas in patients who met the other eligibility criteria of the Parma study, although it is important to note that a majority of the patients ultimately dying of aggressive lymphoma would not meet the eligibility criteria of the Parma study. This study did, however, also raise the question of whether the earlier use of high-dose therapy in untreated patients would prove to be beneficial. Recent data suggest an alternative salvage regimen to DHAP in relapsed or refractory lymphoma, in preparation for high-dose therapy and stem cell transplant. Investigators from Memorial Sloan-Kettering Cancer Center reported on ifosfamide administered as an infusion with bolus carboplatin and etoposide (ICE), supported by G-CSF, given every two weeks for three cycles (median 5.5 weeks), as a shorter regimen, and with a higher overall response rate of 66% than might be expected with DHAP.[41] However, these authors do not report their baseline IPI index at relapse, as did the authors of the Parma trial, where response to DHAP varied significantly by IPI: overall response rates to two courses of DHAP were 77%, 54%, 55%, and 42% in patients with an IPI of 0, 1, 2, and 3, respectively ($p < 0.02$).[40] Unfortunately, in relapsed or primary refractory NHL patients, the Memorial Sloan-Kettering group also report limited benefit in high-risk IPI from their (ICE) salvage followed by high-dose therapy and stem cell transplantation, even in patients with chemosensitive disease: IPI 1 or 2 versus 3 or 4 separated patients into two distinct prognostic groups with 59% versus 20% 2.5-year failure-free survival rate ($p = 0.04$).[42] These authors conclude that new approaches to therapy are needed for these high IPI index relapsed/refractory patients.

In contrast, IPI high-risk DLCL at initial diagnosis, but not lower-risk groups, may benefit from high-dose chemotherapy and stem cell support. The Groupe d'Etudes des Lymphomes des l'Adulte (GELA) reported an important study on a subset of 727 patients treated with the LNH87 protocol. In this study, 370 patients were randomized, after achieving a complete response with standard full-course induction therapy, to consolidation treatment with either sequential chemotherapy or autologous bone marrow transplantation (ABMT). Only one patient died of transplant related complications. With a median follow-up of 21 months, the overall two-year survival rate was 62% and the disease-free survival rate was 58%. Overall survival and disease-free survival for all the randomized patients did not differ between the consolidation arms ($p = 0.089$). This trial was instituted before the publication of the IPI. Therefore, patients were not initially stratified by IPI as an important prognostic factor. A subsequent retrospective analysis did reveal a relapse-free and overall survival benefit for the patients who were reclassified as having the high-intermediate-risk and high-risk characteristics according to the IPI.[43] In another study, Santini and colleagues[44] randomized patients to receive either standard VACOP-B chemotherapy or VACOP-B followed by ABMT (VACOP-B is similar to MACOP-B, but with etoposide instead of methotrexate/leucovorin). While there was no difference in the disease-free survival (DFS) or progression-free survival (PFS) for the entire group of 124 patients; there was a statistical improvement in DFS ($p = 0.008$) and a favorable trend in PFS ($p = 0.08$) for the high-intermediate-risk and high-risk IPI groups assigned to high-dose therapy. Once again, since the high-risk patients were not initially identified as the target population for that trial, prospective randomized trials will clearly be required to determine whether this subset of patients truly benefits from high-dose therapy. Several recent reviews have highlighted the fact that the role of high-dose therapy as primary therapy in high-risk NHL patients is not yet defined, and conclusions await randomized phase III trials.[45,46] The data supports the hypothesis that high-intermediate-risk and high-risk patients with aggressive lymphoma who receive full-course standard induction therapy will benefit from the addition of high-dose therapy. Based on this hypothesis, the Lymphoma Committees and the Bone Marrow Transplant Committees of SWOG have agreed to jointly conduct a randomized clinical trial of early versus delayed high-dose therapy for patients with high-intermediate-risk and high-risk large cell NHL (SWOG 9704). If this study confirms the benefit of high dose therapy in this patient group, subsequent trials will attempt to increase the number of responding patients who become eligible for high-dose therapy.

The use of high-dose therapy is not without risk, and this highlights concern for its use as upfront therapy in NHL. A recent report from the Dana-Farber Cancer Institute describes the incidence of myelodysplasia (MDS) after ABMT.[47] All 552 patients in this study were treated with a uniform regimen, and 41 developed MDS at a median of 47 months after ABMT for NHL. The incidence of MDS was 7.4%, the actuarial incidence at 10 years was 19.8%, and, of most concern, there was no evidence of a plateau. All these issues were raised in the report of the Second International Consensus Conference on High-dose Therapy with Stem Cell Support (HDT).[48] The consensus opinion of this group was that first or subsequent chemosensitive relapse of NHL was the best setting for comparing new regimens in HDT, or the use of autologous versus allogeneic stem cells in HDT. There was no clear consensus in the use of HDT for newly diagnosed NHL patients, because of the lack of availability of results from ongoing randomized trials for poor-prognosis patients.

It is generally understood that the therapeutic benefit of allogeneic bone marrow transplantation is due largely to an immune graft-versus-malignancy effect. This concept has recently been explored in a new procedure in several hematologic malignancies, including NHL. The procedure is termed non-myeloablative stem cell transplantation (NST) or simply nonmyeloablative transplantation.[49,50] NST consists of immunosuppression, followed by infusion of mobilized blood stem cells from siblings (single-locus-mismatched allowed) or marrow cells from matched unrelated donors (MUD) to establish host-versus-graft chimerism and tolerance, with additional immunosuppression by low-dose cyclosporine A (CSA). Persistent evidence of disease or recurrent disease in mixed chimeras is treated by discontinuation of CSA, or by graded increments of donor lymphocyte infusion (DLI). No one is yet sure what regimens give the best chance for engraftment and chimerism. The procedure can be offered to older patients who otherwise would not qualify for allogeneic transplantation. Graft-versus-host disease remains the single major problem.

CONCLUSIONS AND FUTURE DIRECTIONS

History has taught us that prospective randomized clinical trials are only successful when they are based on positive leads provided by solid phase II trials. However, the application of this concept is not always straightforward. In the past, many of the promising phase II studies in DLCL have appeared to be beneficial based on patient selection criteria and not the therapeutic result. The new prognostic factor index now allows us to evaluate the expected therapeutic results based on the mixture of patient risk categories. CHOP has remained the standard treatment for DLCL for over 20 years, but its benefit is limited. It is time to improve. Multiple rationale strategies are now being explored. We believe that improved application of monoclonal antibody therapy in combination with CHOP may advance therapy, if molecular remissions in DLCL have clinical benefit. Continued investigation of high-dose therapy in relapsed and primary refractory disease may advance our treatment of this condition. Progress in the application of nonmyeloablative stem cell transplantation in IPI high-risk relapsed and primary refractory disease may yet yield benefit for this poor-prognosis category. We believe that as our understanding of the molecular biology of NHL improves, and our ability to manipulate genes translates from the bench to the clinic, molecular targets will become the focus of many therapeutic trials. Thoughtful clinical investigation is the key to future progress in NHL.

REFERENCES

1. Greenlee RT, Murray T, Bolden S, Wingo PA, Cancer Statistics, 2000. *CA Cancer J Clin* 2000; **50**: 7–33.

2. The Non-Hodgkin's Lymphoma Pathologic Classification Project, National Cancer Institute sponsored study of classifications of non-Hodgkin's lymphomas: summary and description of a working formulation for clinical usage. *Cancer* 1982; **49**: 2112–35.

3. Harris NL, Jaffe ES, Stein H et al, A revised European–American classifica-

tion of lymphoid neoplasms: a proposal from the International Lymphoma Study Group. *Blood* 1994; **84**: 1361–92.

4. The Non-Hodgkin's Lymphoma Classification Project, A clinical evaluation of the International Lymphoma Study Group classification of non-Hodgkin's lymphoma. *Blood* 1997; **89**: 3909.

5. Jaffe ES, Harris NL, Diebold J, Muller-Hermelink HK, World Health Organization classification of neoplastic diseases of the hematopoietic and lymphoid tissues. A progress report. *Am J Clin Pathol* 1999; **111**(1 Suppl 1): S8–12.

6. Fisher RI, Gaynor ER, Dahlberg S et al, Comparison of a standard regimen (CHOP) with three intensive chemotherapy regimens for advanced non-Hodgkin's lymphoma. *N Engl J Med* 1993; **328**: 1002–6.

7. The International Non-Hodgkin's Lymphoma Prognostic Factors Project, A predictive model for aggressive non-Hodgkin's lymphoma. *N Engl J Med* 1993; **329**: 987–94.

8. Fisher RI, DeVita VT Jr, Hubbard SM et al, Randomized trial of ProMACE-MOPP vs. ProMACE-CytaBOM in previously untreated, advanced stage, diffuse aggressive lymphomas. *Proc Am Soc Clin Oncol* 1984; **3**: 242.

9. Klein U, Goossens T, Fischer M et al, Somatic hypermutation in normal and transformed human B cells. *Immunol Rev* 1998; **162**: 261–80.

10. Vaux DL, Cory S, Adams JM, Bcl-2 gene promotes haemopoietic cell survival and cooperates with c-myc to immortalize pre-B cells. *Nature* 1988; **335**: 440–2.

11. Strasser A, Whittingham S, Vaux DL et al, Enforced BCL-2 expression in B-lymphoid cells prolongs antibody responses and elicits autoimmune disease. *Proc Natl Acad Sci USA* 1991; **88**: 8661–5.

12. Lo Coco F, Ye BH, Lista F et al, Rearrangement of the BCL-6 gene in diffuse large-cell lymphoma. *Blood* 1994; **83**: 1757–9.

13. Ye BH, Lista F, Lo Coco F et al, Alterations of a zinc finger-encoding gene, BCL-6, in large-cell lymphoma. *Science* 1993; **262**: 747–50.

14. Chang CC, Ye BH, Chaganti RS, Dalla-Ferva R, BCL-6 a POZ/zinc-finger protein, is a sequence-specific transcriptional repressor. *Proc Natl Acad Sci USA* 1996; **93**: 6947–52.

15. Dent AL, Shaffer AL, Yu X et al, Control of inflammation, cytokine expression, and germinal center formation by BCL-6. *Science* 1997; **276**: 589–92.

16. Askew DS, Ashumn RA, Simmons BC, Cleveland JL, Constitutive c-myc expression in an IL-3-dependent myeloid cell line suppresses cell cycle arrest and accelerates apoptosis. *Oncogene* 1991; **6**: 1915–22.

17. Gascoyne RD, Adomat SA, Krajewski S et al, Prognostic significance of Bcl-2 protein expression and *bcl*-2 gene rearrangement in diffuse aggressive non-Hodgkin's lymphoma. *Blood* 1997; **90**: 244.

18. Hermine O, Haioun C, Lepage E et al, Prognostic significance of bcl-2 protein expression in aggressive non-Hodgkin's lymphoma. Groupe d'Etude des Lymphomes de l'Adulte (GELA). *Blood* 1996; **87**: 265.

19. Koduru PR, Raju K, Vadmal V et al, Correlation between mutation in p53, p53 expression, cytogenetics, histologic type, and survival in patients with B-cell non-Hodgkin's lymphoma. *Blood* 1997; **90**: 4078–91.

20. Ichikawa A, Kinoshita T, Watanabe T et al, Mutations of the p53 gene as a prognostic factor in aggressive B-cell lymphoma. *N Engl J Med* 1997; **337**: 529–34.

21. Harris NL, Jaffe ES, Diebold J et al, The World Health Organization classification of neoplastic diseases of the hematopoietic and lymphoid tissues. Report of the Clinical Advisory Committee meeting, Airlie House, Virginia, November, 1997. *Ann Oncol* 1999; **10**: 1419–32.

22. Suster S, Primary large-cell lymphomas of the mediastinum. *Semin Diagn Pathol* 1999; **16**: 51–64.

23. Abou-Elella AA, Weisenburger DD, Vose JM et al, Primary mediastinal large B-cell lymphoma: a clinicopathologic study of 43 patients from the Nebraska Lymphoma Study Group. *J Clin Oncol* 1999; **17**: 784–90.

24. Baars JW, de Jong D, Willemse EM et al, Diffuse large B-cell non-Hodgkin lymphomas: the clinical relevance of histological subclassification. *Br J Cancer* 1999; **79**: 1770–6.

25. Ansell SM, Kurtin PJ, Stenson M et al, Evaluation of the proliferative index as a prognostic factor in diffuse large cell lymphoma: correlation with the International Index. *Leuk Lymphoma* 1999; **34**: 529–37.

26. Korsmeyer SJ, BCL-2 gene family and the regulation of programmed cell death. *Cancer Res* 1999; **59**: 1693s–700s.

27. Kodera T, Kohno T, Takakura S et al, Microsatellite instability in lymphoid leukemia and lymphoma cell lines but not in myeloid leukemia cell lines. *Genes Chromosomes Cancer* 1999; **26**: 267–9.

28. Rizzo P, Carbone M, Fisher SG et al, Simian virus 40 is present in most United States human mesotheliomas, but it is rarely present in non-Hodgkin's lymphoma. *Chest* 1999; **116**(6 Suppl): 470S–3S.

29. Cheson BD, Horning SJ, Coiffier B et al, Report of an international workshop to standardize response criteria for non-Hodgkin's lymphomas. *J Clin Oncol* 1999; **17**: 1244.

30. Wilson WH, Little R, Pearson D et al, Phase II and dose-escalation with or without granulocyte colony-stimulating factor study of 9-aminocamptothecin in relapsed and refractory lymphomas. *J Clin Oncol* 1998; **16**: 2345–51.

31. Rosen LS, Irinotecan in lymphoma, leukemia, and breast, pancreatic, ovarian, and small-cell lung cancers. *Oncology* 1998; **12**(8 Suppl 6): 103–9.

32. Sakai C, Saotome T, Takeshita A et al, Improvement of quality of life (QOL) and life prolongation by CPT-11 + Adriamycin (ADM) therapy: report of 4 cases of non-Hodgkin's lymphoma refractory to conventional chemotherapies. *Gan To Kagaku Ryoho* 1999; **26**: 709–14.

33. Zhu XH, Shen YL, Jing YK et al, Apoptosis and growth inhibition in malignant lymphocytes after treatment with arsenic trioxide at clinically achievable concentrations. *J Natl Cancer Inst* 1999; **91**: 772–8.

34. Adams J, Palombella VJ, Sausville EA et al, Proteasome inhibitors: a novel class of potent and effective antitumor agents. *Cancer Res* 1999; **59**: 2615–22.

35. Shipp MA, Neuberg D, Janicek M et al, High-dose CHOP as initial therapy for patients with poor-prognosis aggressive non-Hodgkin's lymphoma: a dose-finding pilot study. *J Clin Oncol* 1995; **13**: 2916–23.

36. Coiffier B, Haioun C, Ketterer N et al, Rituximab (anti-CD20 monoclonal antibody) for the treatment of patients with relapsing or refractory aggressive lymphoma: a multicenter phase II study. *Blood* 1998; **92**: 1927–32.

37. Winkler U, Schulz HR, Klein TO et al, treatment of patients with mantle-cell and aggressive B-cell non-Hodgkin's lymphoma using the monoclonal anti-CD20 antibody rituximab (Rituxan™): evaluation of safety and response. *Blood* 1999; **94**(10 Suppl 1): Abst 4419.

38. Czuczman MS, Grillo-Lopez AJ, White CA et al, Treatment of patients with low-grade B-cell lymphoma with the combination of chimeric anti-CD20 monoclonal antibody and CHOP chemotherapy. *J Clin Oncol* 1999; **17**: 268–76.

39. Vose JM, Link BK, Grossbard ML et al, Phase II study of rituximab in combination with CHOP chemotherapy in patients with previously untreated intermediate- or high-grade non-Hodgkin's lymphoma (NHL). *Blood* 1999; **94**(10 Suppl 1): Abst 388.

40. Blay J, Gomez F, Sebban C et al, The International Prognostic Index correlates to survival in patients with aggressive lymphoma in relapse: analysis of the PARMA trial. Parma Group. *Blood* 1998; **92**: 3562–8.

41. Moskowitz CH, Bertino JR, Glassman JR et al, Ifosfamide, carboplatin, and etoposide: a highly effective cytoreduction and peripheral-blood progenitor-cell mobilization regimen for transplant-eligible patients with non-Hodgkin's lymphoma. *J Clin Oncol* 1999; **17**: 3776–85.

42. Moskowitz CH, Nimer SD, Glassman JR et al, The International Prognostic Index predicts for outcome following autologous stem cell transplantation in patients with relapsed and primary refractory intermediate-grade lymphoma. *Bone Marrow Transplant* 1999; **23**: 561–7.

43. Haioun C, Lepage E, Gisselbrecht C et al, Benefit of autologous bone marrow transplantation over sequential chemotherapy in poor-risk aggressive non-Hodgkin's lymphoma: updated results of the prospective study LNH87-2. Groupe d'Etude des Lymphomes de l'Adulte. *J Clin Oncol* 1997; **15**: 1131–7.

44. Santini G, Salvagno L, Leoni P et al, VACOP-B versus VACOP-B plus autologous bone marrow transplantation for advanced diffuse non-Hodgkin's lymphoma: results of a prospective randomized trial by the non-Hodgkin's Lymphoma Cooperative Study Group. *J Clin Oncol* 1998; **16**: 2796–802.

45. Morrison VA, Peterson BA, High-dose therapy and transplantation in non-Hodgkin's lymphoma. *Semin Oncol* 1999; **26**: 84–98.

46. Johnston LJ, Horning SJ, Autologous hematopoietic cell transplantation in non-Hodgkin's lymphoma. *Hematol Oncol Clin North Am* 1999; **13**: 889–918.

47. Friedberg JW, Neuberg D, Stone RM et al, Outcome in patients with myelodysplastic syndrome after autologous bone marrow transplantation for non-Hodgkin's lymphoma. *J Clin Oncol* 1999; **17**: 3128–35.

48. Shipp MA, Abeloff MD, Antman KH et al, International Consensus Conference on High-Dose Therapy with Hematopoietic Stem Cell Transplantation in Aggressive Non-Hodgkin's Lymphomas: report of the jury. *J Clin Oncol* 1999; **17**: 423–9.

49. Champlin R, Khouri I, Komblau S et al, Reinventing bone marrow transplantation. Nonmyeloablative preparative regimens and induction of graft-vs-malignancy effect. *Oncology* 1999; **13**: 621–8.

50. Slavin S, Nagler A, Naparstek E et al, Well-tolerated non-myeloablative fludaribine-based protocols for the treatment of malignant and non-malignant disorders with allogeneic bone marrow or blood stem cell transplantation. *Blood* **94**(10 Suppl 1): Abst 1562.

7
Extranodal lymphomas

Emanuele Zucca, Annarita Conconi

INTRODUCTION

At least one-quarter of non-Hodgkin's lymphomas (NHLs) arise from tissue other than lymph nodes and even from sites that normally contain no lymphoid tissue. These forms are referred to as primary extranodal lymphomas. Since these tumours, numerous when considered together, are widely distributed throughout the body, it is difficult to find adequate series of any given site.[1,2] Moreover, many historical series were published before the recognition of mucosa-associated lymphoid tissue as the origin of many extranodal lymphomas, and, in general, classification of primary extranodal lymphomas was similar to that of nodal lymphomas, without consideration that their origin could be different. Hence the literature lacks uniformity in histopathological classification. The first attempt to eliminate this problem was made only in 1994 with the proposal of the REAL classification.[3]

There are great differences in the incidence of extranodal lymphomas among countries: USA 24%, Canada 27%, Israel 36%, Lebanon 44%, Denmark 37%, the Netherlands 41%, Italy 48%, and Hong Kong 29% (Table 7.1). Little is known about the actual incidence in developing countries, which, however, seem to have a high incidence of extranodal forms. It has recently been demonstrated that the incidence of NHLs is clearly increasing, and during the past 20 years extranodal disease increased more rapidly than nodal disease. Extranodal lymphomas can arise in almost every organ; the greatest increases have been observed for lymphomas of the central nervous system (CNS), followed by lymphomas of the gastrointestinal (GI) tract and the skin. In addition to the AIDS epidemic, other predisposing factors, such as other viral infections, immunosuppressive treatments, or environmental factors, might explain the increased incidence of extranodal lymphomas.[1]

Signs and symptoms at presentation depend largely on the site; the GI localizations represent the most common form of extranodal lymphoma, while other frequent and clinically important sites include the CNS and the skin. Survival rates also vary among all of the specific sites of primary extranodal lymphomas. This is due partially to differences in natural history, but mainly to differences in management strategy, which are related to organ-specific

Table 7.1 Frequencies (%) and sites of extranodal lymphomas in different countries[1]

	USA	The Netherlands[a]	Denmark[a]	Canada[b]	Hong Kong	Pakistan	Egypt	Switzerland
Stomach	24	23	19	—	39	10	10	36
Small intestine	8	5	9	—	24	17	5	11
Waldeyer's ring	14	16	—[c]	19	8	17	22	15
Nose, sinus	2	1	3	—	9	1	<1	
Orbit	2	3	1	4	1	<1	<1	5
Thyroid gland	3	2	5	6	4	—	—	1
Other head and neck sites	2	4	<1	9	1	—	—	3
CNS	2	6	7	10	—	2	1	1
Extradura	—	—	—	2	—	—	—	
Lung, pleura	4	5	5	1	—	—	—	1
Bone	5	3	9	4	4	2	11	3
Soft tissue	9	2	3	5	3	—	—	1
Breast	2	2	1	2	—	—	—	3
Skin (other than mycosis fungoides)	8	2	11	4	3	8	4	6
Testis	1.5	2	3	—	—	12	—	3
Genitourinary tract	0	1	2	4	4	—	6	<1
Gynecologic tract	1	<1	1	1	4	—	—	1

[a] Population-based tumour registry.
[b] Including only stage I and II disease.
[c] Waldeyer's ring and tonsil considered as nodal site.

problems and to the histologic type.[1,2] Testicular and thyroid lymphomas are more often seen in elderly patients, salivary gland and thyroid lymphomas are significantly more common in females, and intestinal and pulmonary lymphomas are more often found in males. Extranodal lymphomas of the stomach and thyroid are more frequently localized, whereas lymphomas of the lungs, bones, and testes are often widespread. With respect to histological classification, aggressive subtypes (usually diffuse large B-cell lymphomas) are predominant in NHL of CNS, testes, bone, liver, and to some extent the stomach. Certain extranodal sites have characteristic patterns of either B-cell disease (e.g. gastric marginal zone lymphoma, MALT type) or T-cell disease (e.g. cutaneous lymphomas, although a subset of cutaneous B-cell lymphomas does exist).

In this chapter, we shall briefly discuss only the general problems posed by the most common or clinically relevant sites, with special attention to the most relevant contributions appeared in the literature during 1999 and the first quarter of 2000.

PRIMARY GASTROINTESTINAL LYMPHOMAS

The GI tract is the most frequently involved extranodal localization in NHL, accounting for approximately 10–15% of all NHL and 30–40% of all extranodal cases. In the Western world, the most common locations are the stomach and the small intestine.[1]

Infection by *Helicobacter pylori* has been cited as an environmental factor of possible aetiologic relevance in those cases of gastric NHL deriving from so-called mucosa-associated lymphoid tissue (MALT).[4] Less epidemiological information is available on intestinal localizations. Patients with coeliac disease have a significantly increased risk of developing the so-called enteropathy-associated T-cell lymphoma (EATCL), and some authors have suggested that adult-onset coelic disease may be itself a form of low-grade lymphoma.[1]

The applicability of the Ann Arbor staging system to gastrointestinal lymphoma has often been questioned, and several alternative staging systems have been proposed.[5] In gastric lymphoma, variations in diagnostic criteria and staging procedures can have important consequences for patient selection, and can preclude meaningful comparison of published series.[5,6] An international survey of 19 centres has recently been performed with the aim of analysing controversies and consensus in the diagnosis, work-up, and treatment of gastric lymphoma. This study, published in 1999, showed that histological criteria varied among pathologists, with a notable influence of the classification system used in the different countries.[6] Moreover, evaluation of the lymphoma distribution in the gastric wall and routine staging of the GI tract differed between groups headed by medical oncologists and those headed by gastroenterologists. This results in basically different patient selections and bias in treatment outcome. Similar effects were recorded for the role of gastric resection and radiotherapy.

Therefore the optimal treatment of gastrointestinal lymphomas remains a very controversial issue, and depends on the histological type and stage of the disease.[1]

Diffuse large cell lymphoma of the GI tract

Advanced gastrointestinal diffuse large cell lymphoma (DLCL) appears to behave in the same manner as other advanced lymphomas, with comparable histology and prognostic factors. The retrospective analysis of two very large series of gastric DLCL have been published, with an accompanying editorial, in the December 1999 issue of the *Annals of Oncology*, discussing the utility of the International Prognostic Index in identifying subsets of patients with different prognoses.[7–9]

Since the publication in 1991 of a prospective study from the French GELA group including more than 700 patients with aggressive lymphomas treated with intensive chemotherapy, which showed no difference in therapy outcome between those patients with an advanced aggressive nodal lymphoma and those patients (approximately 15%) in which the lymphoma was deemed to have primarily arisen in the GI tract, it has generally been accepted that combination chemotherapy is the treatment of choice for patients with locally advanced or disseminated GI lymphomas of aggressive histological type.[10]

The effectiveness of combination chemotherapy in advanced cases of GI lymphomas has led to reconsideration of the role of primary surgery in less advanced cases.[1,11] New approaches have been advocated. It has been suggested from the results of some recent gastric lymphoma series, including the interim analysis of a large prospective multicentre study from Germany,[12] that chemotherapy, sometimes combined with radiotherapy, can be curative and that gastrectomy is redundant. For primary intestinal lymphoma, however, there are as yet no studies that clearly demonstrate that surgery is unnecessary, and combined-modality treatment is widely considered the procedure of choice.[1]

Gastric marginal zone B-cell lymphoma (MALT lymphoma)

Important achievements have been made in the understanding of the molecular events that may have a relevant pathogenetic role. The rearranged genes at the breakpoints of the t(11;18)(q21;q21) translocation, which is present in at least one-third of cases,[13] have been identified and cloned.[14–16] The rearrangement of the apoptosis inhibitor gene *API-2* on 11q21 may result in a survival advantage for MALT lymphoma B-cell clones carrying the recurrent chromosomal translocation t(11;18)(q21;q21).[14] A second non-random translocation, much more rarely detected namely, the t(1;14)(p22;q32), might confer to the tumour an increased capacity of autonomous growth by means of inactivating mutations and overexpression of the *BCL10* gene.[17,18] However, the oncogenetic role of *BCL10* is still controversial and *BCL10* genomic mutations were almost absent in recent large series of NHL that included several cases of extranodal marginal zone B-cell histology.[19,20]

Increasing evidence indicates that eradication of *H. pylori* with antibiotics can be effectively employed as the sole initial treatment of localized gastric MALT lymphoma. An American uncontrolled trial of 34 patients with stage I–II disease showed that the antibiotic efficacy is higher in early lesions: 70% of the cases with diseases confined to the mucosa and submucosa achieved a complete remission (CR), whilst those with locally advanced disease, infiltrating the muscularis mucosae or the serosa or the perigastric lymph nodes, had a significantly lower CR rate (38%).[21] A preliminary response evaluation has also been performed in the first 170 patients with localized low-grade lymphoma of the stomach enrolled in the ongoing international controlled clinical trial LY03 of chlorambucil versus observation after antibiotic therapy, and it confirmed that at least half of the treated cases can achieve a complete histological regression.[22] However, the histologic and endoscopic remission does not necessarily mean a cure: a polymerase chain reaction (PCR) assay for the detection of monoclonal B cells can remain positive in about half of histological CRs, suggesting that *H. pylori* eradication suppresses but does not eradicate the lymphoma clones.[21,23–27]

No treatment guidelines exist for the management of patients after failure with antibiotics or for the subset of cases in which no evidence of *H. pylori* can be found. It has been shown that the chance of a response to antibiotics is dramatically reduced in this latter group.[21] A choice can be made between conventional oncological modalities, including chemotherapy, radiotherapy, and surgery, alone or in combination.[4,28–32] Unfortunately, there are no published randomized studies to help in the decision.

PRIMARY CUTANEOUS LYMPHOMAS

Primary cutaneous lymphomas can be defined as the presence of cutaneous disease alone, with no nodal or systemic lymphoma. They represent a very numerous group of extranodal lymphomas, accounting for approximately 10% of cases.[1] The proper definition of primary cutaneous lymphoma requires a combination of histological, immunological, and clinical data. On this basis, a classification scheme has been proposed by the EORTC cutaneous lymphoma study group.[33] However, the need of an organ-specific classification scheme is still controversial.[34]

Lymphomas of the skin are more often of T-cell type, with mycosis fungoides and Sézary syndrome comprising around 65% of cases. Mycosis fungoides is characterized by epidermotropic band-like infiltrates of small to medium sized and occasionally large T lymphocytes that are CD3$^+$, CD4$^-$, CD45RO$^+$, CD30$^-$, and CD8$^-$. The clinical course is indolent, with slow progression over years from patches to more infiltrate plaques. The five-year survival rate approximates 90%. Nearly all deaths are due to causes other than mycosis fungoides. In a proportion of patients, lymph nodes and internal organs may be involved in the later stages of disease.[35] Since transformation to large T-cell lymphoma may occur, histological follow-up has been advised to prevent clinical progression associated with a worse prognosis.[36] Local therapy (e.g. PUVA or radiotherapy) is preferred as long as the disease remains confined to the skin. Combination chemotherapy can be used in cases with nodal or visceral involvement or widespread disease refractory to skin-targeted treatments.

Sézary syndrome has been considered to be a leukaemic variant of mycosis fungoides, and is defined by the triad of erythroderma, generalized lymphadenopathy, and the presence of neoplastic T cells (Sézary cells) in skin, lymph nodes, and peripheral blood. Histological and immunohistochemical features are similar to those seen in mycosis fungoides. Chemotherapy and extracorporeal photophoresis have been reported to be effective. However, the disease is aggressive, with a median survival of about three years.[35]

Classification of primary cutaneous B-cell lymphomas is particularly controversial. The subtypes follicle centre lymphoma of the head and trunk and immunocytoma of the EORTC classification comprise over 90% of primary cutaneous B-cell lymphomas. This group includes a large percentage of diffuse large cell lymphomas, which, in the scalp and in the trunk, despite their aggressive cytological and histological features, spread only very rarely beyond the skin and have a clinically indolent course.[37] More aggressive is the clinical course of primary cutaneous large B-cell lymphoma of the leg. Extranodal marginal zone B-cell lymphomas of the skin have also been described; according to some authors, the cutaneous immunocytoma of the EORTC scheme can also be interpreted as a cutaneous marginal zone B-cell lymphoma.[1] Since skin-associated lymphoid tissue (SALT) is usually devoid of B cells, analogous to the MALT concept in the stomach, acquired SALT could represent the background for the development of the lymphoma. Furthermore, the association of cutaneous B-cell lymphoma with acrodermatitis chronica atrophicans suggests that *Borrelia burgdorferi* might have a role similar to that of *H. pylori* in the stomach. Interestingly, regression of cases of cutaneous marginal zone B-cell lymphomas has recently been reported following anti-*B. burgdorferi* antibiotic therapy, but the validity of this new approach has still to be confirmed.[38]

In general, localized cutaneous B-cell lymphomas can be successfully treated with radiation therapy alone, with chemotherapy being reserved for patients with multiple cutaneous or subcutaneous localizations or with diffuse large-cell lymphoma of the legs.

PRIMARY CENTRAL NERVOUS SYSTEM LYMPHOMA

Primary CNS lymphoma (PCNSL) is a disease distinct from other extranodal lymphomas in its biology, clinical features, and response to treatment. PCNSL can be defined as a lymphoma arising in and confined to the cranial–spinal axis (brain, eye, leptomeninges, and spinal cord). In the last decade, PCNSL has showed an increasing incidence both in immunocompromised (congenital, acquired, or iatrogenic) high-risk groups and in the general population.[39,40] The clinical and radiological characteristics of the disease in immunocompetent patients are very different from those observed in AIDS-associated patients, in whom PCNSL often presents with an encephalophatic picture. PCNSL accounts for 1–2% of malignant brain tumours and 2–4% of all extranodal lymphomas.[40] In rare instances, PCNSL presents as a localized leptomeningeal disease in the absence of parenchymal brain involvement. Primary ocular lymphoma (i.e. lymphoma restricted to the globe, usually the vitreous, retina, and choroid) is exceedingly rare. Ocular involvement is often bilateral, and more than half of the patients will later develop brain lesions. Secondary involvement of the CNS occurs in 5–30% of cases of systemic NHL.[2]

PCNSL is usually disseminated within the nervous system at diagnosis, in approximately 40–50% of immunocompetent and in nearly 100% of AIDS patients. About 40% of patients have a demonstrable involvement of the spinal fluid and 20% have involvement of the eyes. In addition to the usual procedures, staging requires contrast-enhanced computed tomography (CT) scan and magnetic resonance imaging (MRI) with gadolinium of the brain and orbits, before steroids are started, because of the rapid radiographic disappearance of tumour following the administration of steroids ('ghost tumour') – a peculiar feature of PCNSL, not shared by any other intracranial malignant tumour. An ophthalmological evaluation with split-lamp examination should also be performed. Most typically, PCNSL appears as a mass in the supratentorial white matter. Histological confirmation is mandatory. The vast majority of PCNSLs are of diffuse large B-cell type, but small non-cleaved cell (Burkitt's) histology is not uncommon in immunocompromised patients.

A surgical procedure more extensive than stereotactic biopsy is rarely indicated. Aggressive surgical decompression with partial or gross total removal of the tumour is of no benefit. Historically, whole-brain radiation has been the treatment of choice, but, despite different radiation schedules with good initial responses, over 90% of patients recur in the brain, often in sites remote from the initial ones.[39,40] Systemic dissemination occurs in only 10% of cases. The prognosis for unselected patients with immunocomponent PCNSL treated with radical irradiation alone is very poor, the five-year survival rate being 5–10%, with a median survival of between 12 and 18 months.[39] Because of the poor results obtained with radiation therapy alone, new approaches have been developed. Several trials have reported encouraging results with systemic chemotherapy combined with radiotherapy, with a five year projected overall survival rate of 30–50% and a median survival of 2–3 years. High-dose methotrexate is the single most effective chemotherapeutic agent in this setting.[41] However, multimodality treatment results in delayed cognitive neurotoxicity, especially in older patients. Several single-institution reports have described encouraging results with systemic chemotherapy alone: mounting evidence is rising that initial chemotherapy should be the treatment of choice, with irradiation being reserved for resistant or relapsing disease.[2,42] Neverthe-less, the experience with this strategy is still limited, and only randomized trials will be able to clarify this controversial issue.

OTHER PARTICULAR ENTITIES ARISING AT EXTRANODAL SITES

As stated before, extranodal lymphoma may arise in any organ or tissue. Here we briefly summarize some of the more recent data related to some peculiar situations.

Primary effusion lymphomas

This rare entity occurs predominantly in HIV-seropositive patients and typi-cally presents as lymphomatous effusions (pleural, pericardial, or ascitic), usu-ally without a solid tumour mass. Histological features comprise large B cells or anaplastic cells. DNA sequences from Kaposi's sarcoma-associated herpes-virus/human herpesvirus-8 (KSHV/HHV-8) and from Epstein–Barr virus (EBV) are detectable in tumour cells of the large majority of cases. Prognosis appears to be dismal, and, because of the small numbers of reported cases, no exact treatment rules can be given.[43]

Interesting data concerning the in vitro modulation of apoptosis of herpesvirus-infected lymphoma cells by antiviral association of interferon-α and azidothymidine have recently been reported. These results suggest a possible strategy to improve the therapy of certain herpesvirus-associated lymphomas.[44]

Nasal angiocentric T/NK-cell lymphoma

This entity has been referred to in the past as lethal midline granuloma and, more recently, as angiocentric T/NK-cell nasal lymphoma. It usually presents with a destructive midline facial tumour. These lymphomas, exceedingly rare in Western countries, are relatively common among Asians and Native Ameri-cans of Central and South America. Evidence for a strong association with EBV infection has been reported. Lymphomas with similar characteristics have sometimes been identified at other extranodal sites. The haemophagocytic syn-drome is a common clinical complication, which adversely affects survival in nasal T/NK-cell lymphoma, and EBV probably plays a role in its patho-genesis.[45]

The available literature concerning the treatment of T/NK-cell nasal/nasal-type lymphoma is poor, with some groups using localized radiotherapy alone, and other multiagent chemotherapy with or without additional radiation therapy. Prognosis is usually poor. In a recent series of patients with local-ized (stages I–II) angiocentric lymphoma treated with radiotherapy alone, the high rate of systemic relapses seems to indicate the need for a multimodality treatment approach.[46]

Primary testicular lymphoma

Primary testicular lymphoma represents 1–2% of all NHLs. This entity is chiefly a disease of the elderly, with 85% of the cases occurring in patients older than 60 years, among whom it is the most common testicular tumour. Histologically, almost all cases are diffuse large B-cell lymphomas. Primary testicular lymphoma shows a marked tendency to systemic dissemination and a propensity to metastasize to a variety of unusual extranodal sites.[1]

Several retrospective series, including some recent ones, have confirmed the unique clinical features of this aggressive entity.[1,47,48] Prognosis is often poor; however, encouraging results have been reported in a very small series of low-risk patients treated with a brief chemotherapy programme and prophylactic controlateral scrotal irradiation in stage I or chemotherapy plus locoregional radiotherapy in stage II disease.[49]

The CNS has been reported as frequent site of relapse, and CNS prophylaxis has been recommended in both localized and advanced stages of the disease.[1]

In order to better define the clinical characteristics of this rare and unique entity, and to possibly design a prospective treatment study, the International Extranodal Lymphoma Study Group (IELSG) is presently analysing single-patient data from several retrospective series collected in different institutions. The results should be published in the current year.

Non-gastrointestinal MALT lymphomas

Extranodal marginal zone B-cell lymphomas of MALT type occur most often in the stomach, but have been described in various non-GI locations, such as lung, breast, salivary glands, skin, ocular adnexa, thyroid, urogenital tract, and even the dura.[2] Nevertheless, the study of the clinical features of non-gastric MALT lymphoma has been historically confronted with difficulty in assembling representative series. In the last few months, however, two large series have been published, confirming that this particular clinicopathological entity has a generally good prognosis despite its presentation as a disseminated disease in about one-third of cases.[50,51] There are no firm guidelines for treatment, which, in localized cases, is usually tailored according to the specific site. An IELSG phase II trial is currently ongoing to evaluate the clinical activity and safety of the anti-CD20 monoclonal antibody rituximab.

REFERENCES

1. Zucca E, Roggero E, Bertoni F, Cavalli F, Primary extranodal non-Hodgkin's lymphomas. Part 1: Gastrointestinal, cutaneous and genitourinary lymphomas. *Ann Oncol* 1997; **8**: 727–37.

2. Zucca E, Roggero E, Bertoni F et al, Primary extranodal non-Hodgkin's lymphomas. Part 2: Head and neck, central nervous system and other less common sites. *Ann Oncol* 1999; **8**: 1023–33.

3. Harris NL, Jaffe ES, Stein H et al, A revised European–American classification of lymphoid neoplasms: a proposal from the International Lymphoma Study Group. *Blood* 1994; **84**: 1361–92.

4. Zucca E, Roggero E, Pileri S, B-cell lymphoma of MALT type: a review with special emphasis on diagnostic and management problems of low-grade gastric tumours. *Br J Haematol* 1998; **100**: 3–14.

5. Rohatiner A, Report on a workshop convened to discuss the pathological and staging classifications of gastrointestinal tract lymphoma. *Ann Oncol* 1994; **5**: 397–400.

6. de Jong D, Aleman BM, Taal BG, Boot H, Controversies and consensus in the diagnosis, work-up and treatment of gastric lymphoma: an international survey. *Ann Oncol* 1999; **10**: 275–80.

7. Cortelazzo S, Rossi A, Roggero F et al, Stage-modified international prognostic index effectively predicts clinical outcome of localised primary gastric diffuse large B-cell lymphoma. International Extranodal Lymphoma Study Group. *Ann Oncol* 1999; **10**: 1433–40.

8. Ibrahim EM, Ezzat AA, Raja MA et al, Primary gastric non-Hodgkin's lymphoma: clinical features, management, and prognosis of 185 patients with diffuse large B-cell lymphoma. *Ann Oncol* 1999; **10**: 1441–9.

9. Gospodarowicz M, Individuality versus conformity. Is perfection necessary in staging and prognostic classifications of specific primary extranodal lymphomas? *Ann Oncol* 1999; **10**: 1405–7.

10. Salles G, Herbrecht R, Tilly H et al, Aggressive primary gastrointestinal lymphomas: review of 91 patients treated with the LNH-83 regimen. A study of the GELA. *Am J Med* 1991; **9**: 77–84.

11. Coiffier B, Salles G, Does surgery belong to medical history for gastric lymphoma? *Ann Oncol* 1997; **8**: 419–21.

12. Willich NA, Reinartz G, Horst EJ et al, Operative and conservative management of primary gastric lymphoma: interim results of a German multicenter study. *Int J Radiat Oncol Biol Phys* 2000; **46**: 895–901.

13. Ott G, Katzenberger T, Greiner A et al, The t(11;18)(q21;q21) chromosome translocation is a frequent and specific aberration in low-grade but not high-grade malignant non-Hodgkin's lymphomas of the mucosa-associated lymphoid tissue (MALT-) type. *Cancer Res* 1997; **57**: 3944–8.

14. Dierlamm J, Baens M, Wlodarska I et al, The apoptosis inhibitor gene AP12 and a novel 18q gene, MLT, are recurrently rearranged in the t(11;18)(q21;q21) associated with mucosa-associated lymphoid tissue lymphomas. *Blood* 1999; **93**: 3601–9.

15. Akagi T, Tamura A, Motegi M et al, Molecular cytogenetic delineation of the breakpoint at 18q21.1 in low-grade B-cell lymphoma of mucosa-associated lymphoid tissue. *Genes Chromosomes Cancer* 1999; **24**: 315–21.

16. Stoffel A, Rao PH, Louie DC et al, Chromosome 18 breakpoint in t(11;18)(q21;q21) translocation associated with MALT lymphoma is proximal to BCL2 and distal to DCC. *Genes Chromosomes Cancer* 1999; **24**: 156–9.

17. Willis TG, Jadayel DM, Du MQ et al, Bcl10 is involved in t(1;14)(p22;q32) of MALT B cell lymphoma and mutated in multiple tumour types. *Cell* 1999; **96**: 35–45.

18. Zhang Q, Siebert R, Yan M et al, Inactivating mutations and overexpression of BCL10 a caspase recruitment

domain-containing gene, in MALT lymphoma with t(1;14)(p22;q32). *Nature Genet* 1999; **22**: 63–8.

19. Luminari S, Intini D, Baldini L et al, Analysis of BCL10 gene mutations in lymphoid malignancies. *Leukemia* 2000; **14**: 905–8.

20. Fakruddin JM, Chaganti RS, Murty VV, Lack of BCL10 mutations in germ cell tumors and B cell lymphomas. *Cell* 1999; **97**: 683–4.

21. Steinbach G, Ford R, Glober G et al, Antibiotic treatment of gastric lymphoma of mucosa-associated lymphoid tissue. An uncontrolled trial. *Ann Intern Med* 1999; **131**: 88–95.

22. Zucca E, Roggero E, Traulle C et al, Early interim report of the LY03 randomised cooperative trial of observation vs chlorambucil after anti-Helicobacter therapy in low-grade gastric lymphoma. *Ann Oncol* 1999; **10**(Suppl 3): 25.

23. Neubauer A, Thiede C, Morgner A et al, Cure of *Helicobacter pylori* infection and duration of remission of low-grade gastric mucosa-associated lymphoid tissue lymphoma. *J Natl Cancer Inst* 1997; **89**: 1350–5.

24. Savio A, Franzin G, Wotherspoon AC et al, Diagnosis and posttreatment follow-up of *Helicobacter pylori*-positive gastric lymphoma of mucosa-associated lymphoid tissue: histology, polymerase chain reaction, or both? *Blood* 1996; **87**: 1255–60.

25. Isaacson P, Gastric MALT lymphoma: from concept to cure. *Ann Oncol* 1999; **10**: 637–45.

26. Press O, Non-Hodgkin's lymphoma. In *American Society of Clinical Oncology. 35th Annual Meeting Summaries* (Johnson D, Whippen D, eds). Baltimore: Lippincott Williams & Wilkins, 1999: 79–82.

27. Isaacson PG, Diss TC, Wotherspoon AC et al, Long-term follow-up of gastric MALT lymphoma treated by eradication of *H. pylori* with antibodies *Gastroenterology* 1999; **117**: 750–1.

28. Hammel P, Haioun C, Chaumette MT et al, Efficacy of single-agent chemotherapy in low-grade B-cell mucosa-associated lymphoid tissue lymphoma with prominent gastric expression. *J Clin Oncol* 1995; **13**: 2524–9.

29. Pinotti G, Zucca E, Roggero E et al, Clinical features, treatment and outcome in a series of 93 patients with low-grade gastric MALT lymphoma. *Leuk Lymphoma* 1997; **26**: 527–37.

30. Schechter NR, Portlock CS, Yahalom J, Treatment of mucosa-associated lymphoid tissue lymphoma of the stomach with radiation alone. *J Clin Oncol* 1998; **16**: 1916–21.

31. Fung CY, Grossbard ML, Linggood RM et al, Mucosa-associated lymphoid tissue lymphoma of the stomach: long term outcome after local treatment. *Cancer* 1999; **85**: 9–17.

32. Schechter NR, Yahalom J, Low-grade MALT lymphoma of the stomach: a review of treatment options. *Int J Radiat Oncol Biol Phys* 2000; **46**: 1093–103.

33. Willemze R, Kerl H, Sterry W et al, EORTC classification for primary cutaneous lymphomas: a proposal from the Cutaneous Lymphoma Study Group of the European Organization for Research and Treatment of Cancer. *Blood* 1997; **90**: 354–71.

34. Jaffe ES, Sander CA, Flaig MJ, Cutaneous lymphomas: a proposal for a unified approach to classification using the REAL/WHO Classification. *Ann Oncol* 2000; **11**(Suppl 1): 17–21.

35. Diamandidou E, Cohen PR, Kurzrock R, Mycosis fungoides and Sézary syndrome. *Blood* 1996; **88**: 2385–409.

36. Vergier B, de Muret A, Beylot-Barry M et al, Transformation of mycosis fungoides: clinicopathological and prognostic features of 45 cases. *Blood* 2000; **95**: 2212–18.

37. Kerl H, Cerroni L, Primary B-cell lymphoma of the skin. *Ann Oncol* 1997; **8**(Suppl 2): 529–32.

38. Roggero E, Zucca E, Mainetti C et al, Eradication of *Borrelia burgdorferi* infection in primary marginal zone B-cell lymphoma of the skin. *Hum Pathol* 2000; **31**: 263–8.

39. De Angelis LM, Yahalom J, Primary central nervous system lymphoma. In: *Cancer: Principles and Practice of Oncology*, 5th edn (De Vita VT Jr, Hellman S, Rosenberg SA, eds). Philadelphia: Lippincott-Raven, 1997: 2233–42.

40. Fine HA, Loeffler JS, Primary central nervous system lymphoma. In: *The Lymphomas* (Canellos GP, Lister TA, Sklar JL, eds). Philadelphia: WB Saunders, 1998; 481–94.

41. O'Brien P, Roos D, Pratt G et al, Phase II multicentric study of brief single-agent methotrexate followed by irradiation in primary CNS lymphoma. *J Clin Oncol* 2000; **18**: 519–26.

42. Schultz C, Scott C, Sherman W et al, Preirradiation chemotherapy with cyclophosphamide, doxorubicin, vincristine, and dexamethasone for primary CNS lymphomas: initial report of Radiation Therapy Oncology Group Protocol 88–06. *J Clin Oncol* 1996; **14**: 556–64.

43. Nador RG, Cesarman E, Chadburn A et al, Primary effusion lymphoma: a distinct clinicopathologic entity associated with the Kaposi's sarcoma-associated herpes virus. *Blood* 1996; **88**: 645–56.

44. Lee RK, Cai JP, Deyev V et al, Azidothymidine and interferon-alfa induce apoptosis in herpesvirus-associated lymphomas. *Cancer Res* 1999; **59**: 5514–20.

45. Jaffe ES, Chan JKC, Su IJ et al, Report of the workshop on nasal and related extranodal angiocentric T/natural killer cell lymphomas. Definitions, differential diagnosis, and epidemiology. *Am J Surg Pathol* 1996; **20**: 103–11.

46. Kim GE, Cho JH, Yang WI et al, Angiocentric lymphoma of the head and neck: patterns of systemic failure radiation treatment. *J Clin Oncol* 2000; **18**: 54–63.

47. Fonseca R, Habermann TM, Colgan JP et al, Testicular lymphoma is associated with a high incidence of extranodal recurrence. *Cancer* 2000; **88**: 154–61.

48. Tondini C, Ferreri AJM, Siracusano L et al, Diffuse large lymphoma of the testis. *J Clin Oncol* 1999; **17**: 2854–8.

49. Connors JM, Klimo P, Voss N et al, Testicular lymphoma: improved outcome with early brief chemotherapy. *J Clin Oncol* 1988; **6**: 776–81.

50. Zinzani PL, Magagnoli M, Galieni P et al, Nongastrointestinal low-grade mucosa-associated lymphoid tissue lymphoma: analysis of 75 patients. *J Clin Oncol* 1999; **17**: 1254–8.

51. Thieblemont C, Berger F, Dumontet C et al, Mucosa-associated lymphoid tissue lymphoma is a disseminated disease in one third of 158 patients. *Blood* 2000; **95**: 802–6.

8
Lymphomas in children

Ian Magrath

INTRODUCTION

In the last 50 years, we have moved from an era in which there was no real expectation of cure, except in the very rare patient with localized disease amenable to locoregional therapy, to cure rates of approximately 90% in childhood lymphomas, including both Hodgkin's and non-Hodgkin's lymphomas (NHL). This is a result of the use of systemic chemotherapy, and its development from single-agent therapy, which resulted in the cure of perhaps 20% of African children with Burkitt's lymphoma in the 1960s, to the intensive drug combinations used in affluent nations today. This result must be close to the peak of what is possible with conventional chemotherapy, and a major focus of the most recently implemented clinical trials has therefore been to attempt to reduce toxicity, both immediate and late, while maintaining the exceptionally good cure rates. Because of the relative rarity of childhood lymphomas, even clinical trials conducted by large cooperative groups require several years to accrue sufficient patient numbers and for follow-up to be sufficient for progression-free survival rates to be meaningful. Thus, international cooperation is likely to speed up the collection of valid information. In this respect, the ongoing collaborative effort among the French Society of Pediatric Oncology (SFOP), the British Medical Research Council, and the US Childrens Cancer Study Group is worthy of special mention. This trial is devoted to determining whether the highly successful SFOP protocol for children with B-cell lymphomas (including both Burkitt's lymphoma and large B-cell lymphoma) may be reduced in intensity and duration in various risk groups without deleterious consequences. To date, results from this trial are not available, but are anticipated to be at least as good as earlier results reported by the SFOP. Because lymphoblastic lymphoma and anaplastic large cell lymphoma – the other major childhood non-Hodgkin's lymphomas – occur less frequently, the numbers of trials conducted and quantity of data available are less than is the case for the B-cell lymphomas, but the best reported results are similar to those achieved with the B-cell lymphomas.

Clearly, empirical clinical trials have paid enormous dividends in the treatment of childhood NHL, but to date, there is little information available regarding the pathogenesis of these diseases – information that could lead to effective strategies to prevent childhood NHL – with the exception of the marked increase in incidence in children with immunodeficiency syndromes, although the lymphomas that occur in this setting differ in many respects from those that occur in children without an underlying disease.

EPIDEMIOLOGY

It has never been clear as to how much the AIDS epidemic in central Africa has influenced the incidence of Burkitt's lymphoma (BL) in children. Many children infected with HIV, of course, die very soon after birth, perhaps before they can develop BL. However, interestingly enough, in Uganda, where the AIDS epidemic has now passed its peak, there has been a recent increase in the incidence of BL.[1] What accounts for this is unclear. In Zimbabwe, where the epidemic is still evolving, there has also been an increase in the incidence of NHL, but particularly in women.[2] The incidence of NHL in children has also been reportedly on the increase in nine European countries, but in children aged 0–14 years between 1970–1990 the overall annual change in incidence was small – an increase of 0.76% annually.[3] This is much less than the reported increase in incidence in adults – perhaps because exposure to environmental agents in the latter is more intensive and more prolonged.

POPULATION-BASED SURVIVAL RATES

The ultimate test of progress in therapy is to determine whether survival at a population level has improved. This is certainly true in USA SEER data, where five-year relative survival rates for NHL in children aged 0–14 years were 77% in 1989–1995 (the latest data available), compared with 44% in 1974–1976. These figures were only slightly higher than for patients aged 0–19 years. In a population-based study of patients registered centrally in Sweden, in which a total of 77 patients were seen over 20 years, Samuelsson et al[4] reported similar figures for the most recent era: a 74% event-free survival rate from 1980 to 1994. This compared with a figure of 19% in the pre-protocol era in Sweden (between 1975 and 1979), clearly demonstrating the importance of therapy in outcome. After treatment, stage and performance status were the next most important factors in determining outcome. Interestingly, in this series, improved survival when Berlin–Frankfurt–Munster (BFM) protocols were used for patients with B-cell lymphomas did not appear to provide an advantage over the LSA_2L_2 protocol, a 10-drug treatment program based on acute lymphoblastic leukemia therapy shown by the US Children's Cancer Study Group in the mid-1980s to be inferior for 'B-Cell' (small non-cleaved cell) lymphomas. The very small number of patients, however, precludes meaningful conclusions in this respect.

B-CELL LYMPHOMAS

Intestinal perforation in children with abdominal NHL is uncommon, but when it does occur is sometimes secondary to attempts to biopsy tumor (tumor-induced perforation is rare, but perforation occasionally occurs post therapy). In a report by Yanchar and Bass,[5] two patients in whom biopsy resulted in perforation died. This report indicates the need to avoid biopsy of tumor in the bowel wall (it is better, where possible, to resect tumor along with a segment of bowel). Laparotomy should also be avoided at the time of presentation, unless required because of an acute abdomen, or because of the absence of tumor outside the abdomen. This applies particularly now that highly effective treatment is available, and surgical resection of intraabdominal tumor is unlikely to be beneficial (one possible exception may be in poor countries, where intensive chemotherapy cannot be given).

One aspect of the good results of treatment of childhood NHL that needs to be addressed is that only a small fraction of patients in the world have access to such therapy. Gradually, highly successful protocols are coming to be used in countries with more limited resources, among the earliest being Eastern European countries. In assessing the results of these transplanted treatment protocols, the possibility of differences in the distribution of biological sub-types and in patients' tolerance of therapy must be born in mind, as well as differences in the analysis of results. In this respect, Kavan et al[6] reported on a series of 63 patients less than 18 years old treated with BFM group protocols in Czech between 1991 and 1995. With the exception of patients with large cell lymphomas, overall results were approximately 10% lower than those reported by the BFM group itself. However, the distribution of cases was atypical, since the majority (22) had large cell lymphoma, and a similar number (19) lymphoblastic lymphoma, while only 10 were reported to have BL. An additional 19 patients with NHL were considered not eligible for the study. Clearly, these results cannot be directly compared with those obtained by the BFM group.

Of particular importance among 1999 publications relating to therapy was a report by the BFM group on the results of therapy in children with B-cell NHL treated in its NHL BFM 90 trial.[7] This study addressed a number of issues raised by the previous BFM trial, NHL BFM 86, as well as by clinical trials conducted by other investigators. One of the important questions asked was whether patients with stage III disease and a serum lactic dehydrogenase (LDH) level of 500 U/L or above – a group that had had a poor prognosis in NHL BFM 86 (43% probability of event-free survival at three years and beyond) – would have an improved probability of event-free survival if treated more intensively. With a tenfold increase in methotrexate dosage from 0.5 g/m^2 to 5.0 g/m^2 being the major change in the therapy of such patients, a markedly improved survival rate was observed in the 90 patients in this subgroup (81% probability of event-free survival; $p = 0.0001$). Whilst this was not a randomized study, and the number of patients in NHL BFM 86 with stage III disease and a serum LDH level of above 500 U/l was not high (23), it is highly probable that this result is valid. Firstly, patients with stage IV disease had a better outcome than stage III patients in the NHL BFM 86 trial – stage IV patients received high-dose methotrexate (5 g/m^2). Secondly, in other published studies, such as the SIOP and NCI studies, in which all stage III patients received more intensive therapy, which included high-dose methotrexate, this poor result in stage III patients with a high LDH level was not observed. It must be stated that 44% of the 90 patients with stage III and LDH ⩾500 U/l received high-dose cytarabine and etoposide because of incomplete tumor resolution after two courses of therapy, and 6.6% of them received autologous bone marrow transplantation because of persistent disease after three courses of therapy. Whether or not these additional treatment elements played a role in the improved outcome of the group as a whole is not clear, but these results, coupled to the finding that LDH was also able to separate higher- and lower-risk patients in both stages III and IV more effectively than stage (indeed, stage IV or the presence of more than 25% of blasts in the bone marrow were not significant factors in a multivariate analysis of stage III, IV, and Burkitt's leukemia patients) are entirely consistent with the long held view that tumor burden (more accurately measured by the surrogate marker, serum LDH, than by stage) is, apart from treatment itself, the most important determinant of outcome. The BFM trial also confirmed that the presence of central nervous system (CNS) disease is not, per se, a poor prognostic sign. Indeed, although patients with CNS disease (26%) had a probability of event-free survival at six years of only 65%, most of the deaths related to the extent of systemic disease (two died of acute tumor cell lysis) or to toxicity (three died of sepsis after a single course of therapy) rather than to CNS disease: only one of the three patients who progressed did so in the CNS. It is of interest that radiation was not a component of the therapy of patients with overt CNS disease – a finding that is also consistent with the growing (and, by many, already accepted) perception that radiation therapy adds nothing but toxicity to children with B-cell lymphomas, regardless of whether or not they involve the CNS. The results of the French–American–British protocol that is examining this question in the context of CNS disease by randomized trial will be awaited with interest, but it will be surprising indeed if radiation proves to be of value. In the BFM study, which included patients with diffuse large B-cell lymphoma, histology was not a prognostic factor, indicating that, whatever their biological differences, large B-cell lymphomas in children are effectively treated by the kind of intensive therapy designed for Burkitt's lymphoma.

These results provide further evidence that high-dose S-phase agents, namely methotrexate and cytarabine, appear to have been pivotal in the management of childhood B-cell NHL – with respect to the treatment of systemic disease as well as CNS disease.

LYMPHOBLASTIC LYMPHOMA

Lymphoblastic lymphoma in childhood also has an excellent prognosis, but, being less common that B-cell lymphomas, there are few data available regarding optimal therapy, particularly in children with limited disease. However, this disease appears to be in a continuum with acute lymphoblastic leukemia, and, in western countries at least, responds well to similar treatment approaches. Amylon and colleagues[8] have examined the hypothesis that high-dose asparaginase consolidation therapy improves survival in pediatric patients with T-cell acute lymphoblastic leukemia or with advanced-stage lymphoblastic lymphoma. There were 195 patients with advanced-stage lymphoblastic lymphoma enrolled in their study, Pediatric Oncology Group (POG) Protocol 8704 (T-3). Patients who achieved a complete remission after intensive induction therapy (90%) were randomized to receive or not receive high-dose intensive asparaginase consolidation: 25 000 IU/m^2 intramuscularly, weekly for 20 weeks. Intrathecal chemotherapy (methotrexate, hydrocortisone, and cytarabine) was given to prevent CNS disease, and CNS irradiation was used only for patients with leukemia and an initial white blood cell count of more than 50 000/μl or patients with active CNS disease at diagnosis. The high-dose asparaginase regimen was significantly superior to the control regimen for both the leukemia and lymphoma subgroups. In lymphoma patients, the four-year continuous remission rate was 78% (standard error (SE) ± 5%) in the high-dose asparaginase-treated group and 64% (SE ± 6%) in the control group ($p = 0.048$). These results confirm the value of asparaginase in lymphoblastic lymphoma of T-cell subtype – indeed, asparaginase is believed to be a particularly valuable element of the BFM protocol, in which an event-free survival rate of 92% has been reported. However, no drug can be considered in isolation, and this result should not be taken as indicating that high-dose asparaginase should be included in all protocols for lymphoblastic lymphoma. In BFM studies, for example, lower doses are given with apparently even better results than those achieved by the POG. The source of asparaginase is another factor that must be taken into consideration, since asparaginase produced by different suppliers varies in its enzymatic activity.

ANAPLASTIC LARGE CELL LYMPHOMA

The very existence of non-random cytogenetic changes associated with specific neoplasms strongly suggests that they have pathogenetic relevance. The observation that a gene is inappropriately expressed by virtue of a non-random chromosomal translocation is a strong argument for the pathogenetic relevance of the gene in question – one that is ultimately confirmed by the development of an understanding of the precise oncogenetic mechanism. Prior to such knowledge, the deregulation of the same gene by several different non-random translocations (as is the case of c-*MYC* in Burkitt's lymphoma or *BCL6* in diffuse large B-cell lymphoma, for example), provides additional evidence for pathogenetic relevance. A number of investigators have now demonstrated that in anaplastic large cell lymphoma (ALCL), inappropriate expression of anaplastic large cell kinase gene, *ALK*, can be brought about by more than one translocation. Rosenwald et al,[9] for example, recently described two new variant translocations in children with ALCL in which ALK protein expression was demonstrated by immunohistochemistry in the absence of a classic t(2;5) translocation. The variant translocations were a t(1;2)(q25;p23) and a t(2;3)(p23;q21). This suggests that genes other than *NPM*, whose product forms a fusion protein with ALK in the t(2;5) translocation, can activate ALK. Interestingly, the ALK proteins expressed in these cases were larger (104 kDa and 97 kDa, respectively) than the ALK expressed in the presence of a t(2;5) translocation. Of additional interest was the observation that ALK expression was confined to the cytoplasm of the tumor cells in the variant cases, in contrast to the more generally observed localization in both nucleus and cytoplasm of NPM–ALK (at least, in the large cells). The significance of this finding remains to be elucidated.

More information is accruing that suggests that, with present treatment approaches, the expression of ALK, which is not invariable in ALCL, is associated with a good prognosis. Indeed, the expression of ALK may well delineate a specific disease entity. Falini et al[10] reported that ALK$^+$ ALCL mostly occurred in children and young adults (mean age, 22 years) in which it usually presented as an aggressive, extensive disease frequently associated with systemic symptoms (75%) and extranodal involvement (60%), especially skin (21%), bone (17%), and soft tissues (17%). ALK$^-$ cases occurred more often in older individuals (mean age 43.33 years), differed with respect to the male-to-female ratio, and were less likely to have advanced or extranodal disease at presentation. Overall survival of patients with ALK$^+$ lymphoma was far better than that of ALK$^-$ large cell lymphoma (71% ± 6% versus 15% ± 11%, respectively). Similar findings were reported by Cataldo et al,[11] who compared fluorescence in situ hybridization (FISH) detection of the t(2;5) translocation with ALK detection by reverse-transcriptase polymerase chain reaction (RT-PCR) in paraffin-embedded tissue, and found no difference in their admittedly small series. Ultimately, immunohistochemistry is likely to prove to be a simpler and more effective means of identifying 'alkomas', and has the advantage over FISH that, with appropriate antibodies, aberrant ALK expression will be detected no matter what the nature of the cytogenetic lesion that led to its production.

Tomaszewski and colleagues[12] described three children with primary ALCL of the skin. At least five more childhood cases of cutaneous ALCL have been reported. Primary cutaneous ALCL is unusual in children, but not uncommon in adults, in whom it is usually associated with a good prognosis and the absence of a t(2;5) translocation. In all three of the cases reported by Tomaszewski et al,[12] the patients developed recurrent disease in the skin at sites separate from the primary location. Chemotherapy did, however, appear to be effective. It should not be assumed that primary cutaneous ALCL in children is the same disease as that observed in adults, and chemotherapy may be the treatment of choice, but information at the present time remains limited.

RARE NON-HODGKIN'S LYMPHOMAS IN CHILDREN

All of the more indolent lymphomas are extremely uncommon in childhood, and follicular lymphoma is no exception. However, Finn et al[13] recently reported four unusual primary follicular lymphomas of the testes in children ranging from 3 to 10 years of age. Three of the four cases were confirmed to be comprised of monoclonal B-cell populations. In contrast to adult follicular lymphomas, none of the four tumors expressed BCL2, nor were *BCL2* gene rearrangements detected in the three cases studied. Surprisingly, BCL6 protein was expressed by all three lymphomas studied, and a *BCL6* gene rearrangement was detected in the one case analyzed by Southern blot. All four boys were treated by orchiectomy and combination chemotherapy, and remained alive without evidence of disease 18–44 months after diagnosis. These neoplasms more closely resemble the large cell (grade 3) type of adult follicular lymphoma, but it is possible that pathogenetic mechanisms differ in the rare childhood lymphomas compared with those that develop in adults.

LYMPHOMAS IN PATIENTS WITH PRIMARY IMMUNODEFICIENCY

Seidemann et al[14] reported on the results of therapy in patients with NHL as a complication of primary immunodeficiency entered into three different BFM trials between October 1986 and April 1997. Of the 1413 patients registered on these studies, 19 had underlying primary immunodeficiency, 6 common variable immunodeficiency, and 13 ataxia telangiectasia. While this study is not truly population-based, since the data have been collected from a large cooperative group, it does provide a reasonable estimate of the fraction of childhood lymphomas that arise in patients with underlying immunodeficiency as well as of the spectrum of lymphomas encountered in such patients. Interestingly, 6 of the lymphomas were of T-cell lineage, the remainder being of B-cell origin, both subtypes of lymphoma occurring in each underlying immunodeficiency state. The distribution of lymphoma subtypes between patients with underlying immunodeficiency and without differed, in that a higher proportion of patients with immunodeficiency (32%) had large B-cell lymphomas and 26% had ALCL (compared with 8% and 11% in non-immunosuppressed patients respectively). Only 21%, compared with 48%, had Burkitt's lymphoma/leukemia. While toxicity encountered was greater in the immunosuppressed patients (3, for example, died of sepsis), 10 patients are in first continuous remission after a median follow-up of four years, indicating that curative attempts at therapy are warranted.

AUTOIMMUNE LYMPHOPROLIFERATIVE SYNDROME

An interesting form of autoimmune disease associated with lymphoprolifera-
tion and often expansion of CD4 and CD8 double-negative T cells has recently
been described. In this disease, mutations of the CD95 (Fas) receptor lead to
defects in Fas-triggered apoptosis and consequent defects in the control of
lymphocyte activation and lymphocyte homeostasis. This syndrome is associated with various clinical manifestations, including lymphoma. Interestingly, a
number of different types of lymphoma have been described, even in the same
family. In one family, reported by Peters et al,[15] for example, both Hodgkin's
disease and T-cell lymphomas were observed. One family member (the
father of the child with T-cell lymphoma) suffered only from a mild hemolytic
anemia.

HODGKIN'S DISEASE

In pediatric Hodgkin's disease, the focus continues to be on reducing therapy
as much as possible whilst retaining the excellent overall survival rates of 90%
or more, which are generally obtained – even in some developing countries.[16]
In children, late effects are particularly important because of the patients' long
potential lifespans. Cardiovascular disease and second malignancies are the
most likely causes of a reduced lifespan in patients who do not develop recurrent Hodgkin's disease, and, in the large Stanford series, account for half of all
deaths in patients treated for Hodgkin's disease.[17] Gervais-Fagnou et al[18] from
Toronto analyzed a series of 427 women, with a mean follow-up of 12.3 years,
which showed that women less than or 30 years of age, after supradiaphragmatic irradiation for Hodgkin's disease, have a 10-fold elevated risk of developing breast cancer compared with the general population – a result which is
entirely consistent with previously published data. In a series of 106 children
at St Jude Children's Research Hospital with stage I and II supradiaphragmatic
Hodgkin's disease treated definitively by irradiation, there was an 11-fold
increased risk of second malignancy and a 68-fold increased risk of fatal cardiac disease (there was also a 33-fold increased risk of infection related to
splenectomy).[19] King et al[20] more precisely documented the frequency of
carotid artery disease in a series of 42 young patients who had had radiation to
the neck for Hodgkin's disease in childhood or young adulthood. Carotid
ultrasonography revealed that approximately a quarter of patients had asymptomatic abnormalities of the carotid artery intima-media. Unless suspected and
dealt with appropriately, this complication could eventually translate into an
increased incidence of stroke. Impaired reproductive function is also a well-
known late effect of treatment for Hodgkin's disease, but is relatively poorly
defined in patients treated as children. Papadakis et al[21] studied 65 patients (36
males and 29 females), who received radiotherapy alone, chemotherapy alone,
or both therapeutic modalities. It was found that all children progressed

through puberty to full sexual maturity, regardless of therapy (including pelvic irradiation in some). Most males had evidence of germinal cell dysfunction but no Leydig cell dysfunction, whilst most females retained normal ovarian function. In some females, hormone levels (FSH and LH), which were abnormally elevated shortly after therapy, returned to normal, and several (6) ultimately delivered healthy babies. Thus, ovarian function in females may recover post chemotherapy, a phenomenon that has also been reported with respect to germ cell function in males.

The German–Austrian Pediatric Hodgkin's Disease Study Group have published the results of their study DAL-HD-90,[22] which was designed in the context of the group's long-term goal of reducing late effects whilst maintaining the excellent results achieved with their earlier regimens OPPA (vincristine, prednisone, procarbazine, and doxorubicin) or OPPA/COPP (where, in the COPP component, cyclophosphamide is given in place of doxorubicin) and involved-field radiotherapy. This group has previously shown that the risk of leukemia is reduced when mechlorethamine is replaced by cyclophosphamide. They have also shown that two cycles of OEPA (vincristine, etoposide, prednisone, and doxorubicin) do not impair testicular function, although additional therapy with COPP does add a negative effect on spermatogenesis, presumably primarily due to procarbazine. In the DAL-HD-90 study, in order to reduce the risk of testicular dysfunction, OEPA was used for the two cycles of induction in boys. Girls continued to be induced with two cycles of OPPA. Patients in treatment groups 2 and 3, with intermediate or advanced stages, received two or four additional cycles, respectively, of COPP, along with low-dose radiation to initially involved sites. Radiation doses and volumes were also further reduced compared with previous treatment protocols. A total of 578 children less than 18 years old (319 boys and 259 girls) were enrolled between 1990 and 1995 and allocated to one of the three treatment arms. Only 8 of the 578 patients had early disease progression, 37 patients relapsed, and there were 3 second malignancies (none of which were leukemias). With a median follow-up of 5.1 years (maximum 8.1 years), 13 patients have so far died, while the probability of five-year event-free survival is 91%, and the overall survival rate is 98% for the entire group. There were no significant differences between the two types of induction therapy. Only preliminary studies of testicular function have been performed, but early results suggest a lower rate of germ cell damage than with the OPPA regimen, and the more limited radiation therapy in this trial did not result in a poorer outcome, even in patients with large mediastinal masses. This begs the question as to the role of radiation in these patients and whether some or even all patients could be treated with chemotherapy alone – a question being asked by many in view of the serious late effects of radiation. Clearly, such an approach would presuppose the use of appropriate chemotherapy regimens with a very low leukemogenic effect (such are possible, as evidenced by the German–Austrian studies, and information from other neoplasms treated with chemotherapy alone), but good clinical trials will need to be performed to study the shortest duration consistent with maintaining the present high event-free survival rates. The incidence of second solid tumors in the German–Austrian studies will be awaited with interest.

In sum, 1999 was a year of confirmation of the excellent results being achieved in the childhood lymphoma, and one in which additional evidence has been accrued that, within each lymphoma subtype, careful stratification of patients for different treatment arms in which the intensity of chemotherapy differs, based on the most accurate markers of tumor burden, permits the toxic cost of therapy to be minimized. The results presently being obtained will be hard to improve upon, at least in terms of survival rates. A small percentage of patients still die, however, from the toxicity of intensive therapy, and it seems probable that while further 'fine-tuning' may still be possible, decreasing toxicity in any major way, as well as salvaging the few remaining patients with resistant disease from the outset (now the two major causes of treatment failure in patients with NHL), awaits the development of more specifically targeted therapies, i.e., therapies directed at the molecular lesions that are the immediate cause of cancer. Such approaches should also result in a reduction in the frequency of late effects.

REFERENCES

1. Parkin DM, Wabinga H, Nambooze S, Wabwire-Mangen F, AIDS-related cancers in Africa: maturation of the epidemic in Uganda. AIDS 1999; 13: 2563–70.

2. Chokunonga E, Levy LM, Bassett MT et al, Aids and cancer in Africa: the evolving epidemic in Zimbabwe. AIDS 1999; 13: 2583–8.

3. Weidmann C, Black RJ, Masuyer E, Parkin DM, Incidence of non-Hodgkin's lymphoma in children between 1970 and 1990 in nine European countries. Eur J Cancer 1999; 35: 1235–7.

4. Samuelsson BO, Ridell B, Rockert L et al, Non-Hodgkin lymphoma in children: a 20-year population-based epidemiologic study in western Sweden. J Pediatr Hematol Oncol 1999; 21: 103–10.

5. Yanchar NL, Bass J, Poor outcome of gastrointestinal perforations associated with childhood abdominal non-Hodgkin's lymphoma. J Pediatr Surg 1999; 34: 1169–74.

6. Kavan P, Kabickova E, Gajdos P et al, Treatment of children and adolescents with non-Hodgkin's lymphoma (results based on the NHL Berlin–Frankfurt–Munster 90 protocols). Cas Lek Cesk 1999; 138: 40–6.

7. Reiter A, Schrappe M, Tiemann M et al, Improved treatment results in childhood B cell neoplasms with tailored intensification of therapy: a report of the Berlin–Frankfurt–Munster group trial NHL-BFM 90. Blood 1999; 94: 3294–306.

8. Amylon MD, Schuster J, Pullen J et al, Intensive high-dose asparaginase consolidation improves survival for pediatric patients with T cell acute lymphoblastic leukemia and advanced stage lymphoblastic lymphoma: a Pediatric Oncology Group study. Leukemia 1999; 13: 335–42.

9. Rosenwald A, Ott G, Pulford K et al, t(1;2)(q21;p23) and t(2;3)(p23;q21): two novel variant translocations of the t(2;5)(p23;q35) in anaplastic large cell lymphoma. Blood 1999; 94: 362–4.

10. Falini B, Pileri S, Zinzani PL, Carbone A et al, ALK + lymphoma: clinicopathological findings and outcome. Blood 1999; 93: 2697–706.

11. Cataldo KA, Jalal SM, Law ME,

Detection of t(2;5) in anaplastic large cell lymphoma: comparison of immunohisto-chemical studies, FISH, and RT-PCR in paraffin-embedded tissue. *Am J Surg Pathol* 1999; **23**: 1386–92.

12. Tomaszewski MM, Moad JC, Lupton GP, Primary cutaneous Ki-1 (CD30) pos-itive anaplastic large cell lymphoma in childhood. *J Am Acad Dermatol* 1999; **40**: 857–61.

13. Finn LS, Viswanatha DS, Belasco JB et al, Primary follicular lymphoma of the testis in childhood. *Cancer* 1999; **85**: 1626–35.

14. Seidemann K, Tiemann M, Henze G et al, Therapy for non-Hodgkin lym-phoma in children with primary immunodeficiency. An analysis of 19 patients from the BFM trials. *Med Pediatr Oncol* 1999; **33**: 536–44.

15. Peters AM, Kohfink B, Martin H et al, Defective apoptosis due to a point mutation in the death domain of CD95 associated with autoimmune lymphopro-liferative syndrome, T-cell lymphoma, and Hodgkin's disease. *Exp Hematol* 1999; **27**: 868–74.

16. Buyukpamukcu M, Atahan L, Caglar M et al, Hodgkin's disease in Turkish children: clinical characteristics and treatment results of 210 patients. *Pediatr Hematol Oncol* 1999; **16**: 119–29.

17. Donaldson SS, Hancock SL, Hoppe RT, The Janeway Lecture. Hodgkin's dis-ease – finding the balance between cure and late effects. *Cancer J Sci Am* 1999; **5**: 325–33.

18. Gervais-Fagnou DD, Girouard C, Laperriere N et al, Breast cancer in women following supradiaphragmatic irradiation for Hodgkin's disease. *Oncol-ogy* 1999; **57**: 224–32.

19. Shah AB, Hudson MM, Poquette CA et al, Long-term follow-up of patients treated with primary radiotherapy for supradiaphragmatic Hodgkin's disease at St. Jude Children's Research Hospital. *Int J Radiat Oncol Biol Phys* 1999; **44**: 867–77.

20. King LJ, Hasnain SN, Webb JA et al, Asymptomatic carotid arterial disease in young patients following neck radiation therapy for Hodgkin lymphoma. *Radiol-ogy* 1999; **213**: 167–72.

21. Papadakis V, Vlachopapadopoulou E, Van Syckle K et al, Gonadal function in young patients successfully treated for Hodgkin disease. *Med Pediatr Oncol* 1999; **32**: 366–72.

22. Schellong G, Potter R, Bramswig J et al, High cure rates and reduced long-term toxicity in pediatric Hodgkin's dis-ease: the German–Austrian multicenter trial DAL-HD-90. The German–Austrian Pediatric Hodgkin's Disease Study Group. *J Clin Oncol* 1999; **17**: 3736–44.

9

AIDS-lymphoma

Daniele Bernardi, Michele Spina, Umberto Tirelli

INTRODUCTION

The aim of this chapter is to critically review all the literature of the year 1999 on HIV-related lymphoid malignancies. To do this, we decided to split our work into two parts: non-Hodgkin's lymphoma (divided into incidence and epidemiology, pathologic and biologic features, and clinical features and therapy) and Hodgkin's disease.

NON-HODGKIN'S LYMPHOMA

Incidence and epidemiology

Since the beginning of the AIDS epidemic, the incidence of non-Hodgkin's lymphoma (NHL) in the USA among HIV-infected individuals is approximately 60 times greater than that expected in the general population – a significant increase.[1] These tumors appear most commonly in the end stages of AIDS, when the immune system is markedly impaired.

Recently the use of highly active antiretroviral therapy (HAART) has been associated with a significant reduction in various opportunistic diseases in HIV-infected patients. The impact of HAART regimens on the incidence of systemic lymphoma remains unclear, but it can be hypothesized that improved immune function and reduced B-cell stimulation in patients receiving HAART may reduce the risk of developing lymphoma. In contrast, however, it is possible that patients treated with HAART may survive longer, with continued B-cell stimulation and dysregulation resulting in an increased incidence of lymphoma over time. Grulich[2] concludes that the incidence rate of AIDS-related NHL has decreased with the use of HAART but that the magnitude of the decrease appears to be less than that for other AIDS-associated opportunistic infections and Kaposi's sarcoma (KS). Possible reasons include the fact that NHL is due to a variety of causes rather than a specific infective agent, the fact that NHL occurs at less profound levels of immune deficiency than most other opportunistic infections, and the B-cell stimulation that occurs in people with AIDS. The favorable impact of HAART may thus be smaller for NHL than for other AIDS-defining illnesses.[3,4] The same conclusion is drawn by Rabkin and co-workers[5] from the AIDS Clinical Trial Group (ACTG), who suggest that while KS incidence has decreased as a concomitant of improved therapy for HIV infection, the smaller change in NHL incidence may be due to the fact that current therapeutic strategies do not eliminate lymphoma risk.

If HAART remains only partly effective in immune system reconstitution, it is likely that NHL will become proportionally more important as a cause of morbidity and mortality in people with HIV and AIDS. This emphasizes the need for HIV treatment strategies that will more completely reverse immune deficiency and immune stimulation. Some other authors[6] have underlined the fact that, in contrast to patients affected by KS, who cease to be at risk of KS once immune function has been improved by antiretroviral therapy, patients with a history of severe immune deficiency continue to be at risk of NHL despite antiretroviral combination therapy.

Although the initiation of carcinogenesis may require an immunodeficient state, the factors promoting the development of NHL further along the causal chain do not seem to be related to immune function – or are related to aspects not affected by any retroviral combination therapy. NHL will thus remain a relatively common complication among patients treated with antiretroviral combination therapy.

Pathologic and biologic features

Although the exact cause of AIDS-related NHL is unknown, various mechanisms seem to play a role in the pathogenesis of the disease. HIV infection leads to chronic B-cell stimulation and proliferation, and ongoing infection by Epstein–Barr virus (EBV) may also promote chronic B-cell proliferation in patients with HIV infection. B-cell proliferation is also known to be induced by monocytes and T cells infected by HIV releasing pro-inflammatory cytokines such as interleukin (IL)-6 and IL-10.[7] Moreover, the incidence of increasing serum levels of IL-10 has been shown to correlate with HIV disease progression, and therapy with HAART results in the gradual decrease, but not elimination, of serum IL-10 level.[8] Constitutive production of high levels of IL-10 has been reported in AIDS-NHL, AIDS pleural effusion lymphomas,[9] AIDS-related Hodgkin's disease, and AIDS central nervous system (CNS) lymphomas. A higher level of IL-6 was found by Crabb Breen et al[10] in the serum of HIV-infected individuals prior to the diagnosis of lymphoma; serum IL-6 was significantly elevated in subjects who developed Burkitt's small non-cleaved cell lymphoma, but not in those subjects who developed large cell, immunoblastic or CNS lymphoma, compared with CD4-matched AIDS controls who did not have lymphoma. The role of chemokines in lymphomagenesis of AIDS has been examined by Rabkin et al[11] and Dean et al,[12] who identified a correlation with the expression of chemokine and chemokine receptor (CCR5 and CCR2) gene variants and risk of developing AIDS-NHL.

The overwhelming majority of cases of systemic AIDS-NHL fall within two main histologic categories: small non-cleaved cell lymphoma (SNCCL), which includes classic Burkitt's lymphoma (BL) and Burkitt-like lymphoma (40%), and diffuse large cell lymphoma (DLCL), which includes large non-cleaved cell lymphoma (LNCCL) (25%), immunoblastic lymphoma plasmocytoid (IBL-P) (25%), and CD30+ anaplastic large B-cell lymphoma (ALCL).

Viral infection of AIDS-BL tumor cells is mainly represented by EBV infection. EBV infection in AIDS-BL, as well as in other AIDS-NHL, is generally monoclonal, consistent with the hypothesis that the virus had been present in the tumor progenitory cell since the early phases of its clonal expansion and thus putatively contributed to lymphoma development. The precise role of EBV in AIDS-BL pathogenesis, however, has remained controversial. Recently, it has been hypothesized that cell transformation in tumors expressing the EBV latency 1 phenotype may be mediated at least in part by a class of non-coding though highly expressed small mRNAs termed Epstein–Barr virus-encoded RNAs (EBERs).[13] Because EBERs are expressed in AIDS-BL, it is possible that these mRNAs play a pathogenetic role in the development and growth of this lymphoma.

The molecular pathogenesis of AIDS-DLCL is more heterogeneous than that of AIDS-BL. In particular, genetic studies performed to date have failed to reveal a common genetic alteration in these lymphomas. Infection by EBV occurs in a significant proportion of cases of AIDS-DLCL. However, only a proportion of infected cases, mainly those categorized as IBL-P, express the EBV-encoded LMP1 protein. It is conceivable that in EBV-infected AIDS-DLCL expressing LMP1, the virus plays the major pathogenetic role.

Curiosity has been raised by Schroeder et al[14,15] about the role of a soluble cytokine (sCD23) that acts as a B-cell growth factor and is associated with EBV infection. In their study, higher levels of serum sCD23 were associated with the absence of tumor EBV and with small non-cleaved cell morphology. Thus, the serum sCD23 level does not appear to be mediated by EBV in these patients, but could be related to a pathogenetic mechanism of small non-cleaved cell lymphoma.

A possible explanation for the frequent extranodal involvement by HIV-NHL has been hypothesized by Chirivi et al:[16] HIV-tat, the transactivating gene product of HIV-1, can enhance the migration of AIDS-related lymphoma cells and their adhesion to endothelial cells. In AIDS patients, this may contribute to the homing and growth of malignant lymphomas at extranodal sites.

Clinical features and therapy

One of the distinguishing features of AIDS-NHL is the widespread extent of the disease at initial presentation and the frequency of systemic B symptoms. At the time of diagnosis, approximately 75% of patients have advanced disease, with frequent involvement of extranodal sites.[17]

Peripheral CNS lymphoma (PCNSL) is a manifestation of very advanced HIV disease; the lymphoma develops as single or multiple lesions in the deep regions of the white matter in the basal ganglia and in the cerebellum. A major clinical problem with PCNSL is its correct identification. When computed tomography (CT) scan or magnetic resonance imaging (MRI) identify an intracranial mass in an HIV-infected individual, the patient is usually first treated with anti-toxoplasmosis treatment, and brain biopsy is considered only after antibiotic failure. To avoid the need for brain biopsy, recent experiences have been done with positron emissions tomography (PET) and thallium single-photon emission CT (SPECT), suggesting that these non-invasive techniques may be able to distinguish tumor from CNS infection and offer the opportunity of a rapid diagnosis. The experience by Antinori et al[18] with a combined approach with thallium SPECT and EBV-DNA detection in cerebrospinal fluid shows a very high diagnostic accuracy in discriminating PCNSL and non-neoplastic focal brain lesions in patients with AIDS. These minimally invasive, easy, and safe diagnostic tools might in some cases represent a valid alternative to invasive procedures, also allowing a better and faster identification of patients requiring brain biopsy. Moreover, in a cost–benefit evaluation, radionuclides and biomolecular technology seem to be less expensive than a standard diagnostic approach, especially when considering surgical procedures and hospitalization time.

The prognosis of HIV-related NHL is poor: the median survival ranges from four to six months in most series. Different factors, including clinical and pathological aggressiveness of the lymphoma, poor clinical conditions of patients, and underlying immunodeficiency, may account for the worse outcome seen in patients with NHL and HIV infection compared with the general population. The optimal treatment for HIV-related NHL remains controversial. The use of intensive combination chemotherapy would be indicated considering the aggressive clinico-pathologic characteristics of lymphoma; however, its toxic side-effects can be prohibitive in HIV-infected patients. Nevertheless, the possibility of obtaining long-term survival and cure with aggressive chemotherapy in a subgroup of patients has been demonstrated clearly, even if the optimal dosage of chemotherapy is still debated.

Given these controversies, the search for prognostic indicators in HIV-related NHL is of total importance in finding the best treatment program. In this setting, the International Prognostic Index (IPI) has been proven to be a reliable prognostic indicator in patients with systemic HIV-related NHL,[19] and it is believed that the IPI system could usefully complement the CD4 cell count as a prognostic indicator in making treatment decisions. The correlation between the degree of immunodeficiency and the IPI may suggest that the severity of immunodeficiency in HIV-positive patients contributes significantly to the aggressive presentation of lymphoma. Patients with higher-risk IPI scores have both high lactate dehydrogenase (LDH) levels and advanced disease stages – two lymphoma-related parameters of IPI that are the hallmarks of high tumor burden and of a tendency of lymphoma toward early dissemination.

Before the introduction of HAART, the median survival of patients with AIDS and NHL who underwent multiagent chemotherapy was 31–35 weeks. This historical survival rate might even be biased, because only patients whose conditions allowed the initiation of multiagent chemotherapy were enrolled in therapeutic trials and thus were reported. In a Swiss retrospective study,[20] a much more favorable survival was found for a subgroup of patients who were treated with full-dose chemotherapy. The Swiss retrospective study suggests that the prognosis may be significantly improved in the era of HAART, which also appears to increase the CD4 cell counts among patients undergoing multiagent chemotherapy. This rise in CD4 cells seems to reflect improved immune function, which can prevent complications associated with chemotherapy for HIV-associated malignancies.

Since HAART would otherwise allow long life expectancy, the high relapse rate of AIDS-NHL represents a novel challenge. Several patients with systemic AIDS-NHL are therefore considered today for second-line chemotherapy. Salvage regimens employed for non-HIV NHL frequently contain moderately high doses of cytotoxic drugs not used during initial therapy, but these protocols may result in profound myelosuppression and immunosuppression in previously treated HIV-positive patients, resulting in significant risk of opportunistic infections and prolonged aplasia. The report from Campbell and co-workers[21] suggests that high-dose chemotherapy followed by peripheral blood stem cell transplantation is a feasible option in selected patients with relapsed HIV-related NHL, given the current improvements in suppression of viral replication and post-transplant supportive care.

HODGKIN'S DISEASE

Patients affected by HIV infection are reported to be at increased risk of Hodgkin's disease (HD). HIV-associated HD shows several peculiarities when compared with HD of the general population. First of all, HIV-HD exhibits an unusually aggressive clinical behavior and is associated with a poor prognosis. Moreover, the pathologic spectrum of HIV-HD differs from that of HD in the general population. In particular, the aggressive histologic subtypes of classic HD, namely mixed cellularity and lymphocyte depletion, predominate among HIV-HD, and tumor tissue is characterized by an unusually large proportion of neoplastic cells termed Reed–Sternberg (RS) cells.

The biologic reasons for the clinico-pathologic peculiarities of HIV-HD are known only in part, and may reflect peculiarities in the tumor microenvironment, as well as in the tumor clone. Carbone and co-workers[22] found that RS cells of all histologic categories of HIV-HD consistently display the $BCL6^-$/syndecan-1^+ phenotype and thus reflect post-germinal center B cells. RS cells of virtually all HIV-HD cases express the EBV-encoded LMP1, which may contribute, at least in part, to modulation of the RS cell phenotype in HIV-HD. According to this model, LMP1 expression, presumably in cooperation with other cellular signals, would induce RS cells to downregulate BCL6, thus allowing further maturation of the tumor clone to assume a post-germinal center phenotype. This model prompts investigations aimed at dissecting the signaling cascade mediated by LMP1 in the context of HIV-HD and at defining the precise pathway exploited for the modulation of RS cell phenotype in hosts infected with HIV.

One of the most peculiar features of HIV-related HD is the widespread extent of the disease at presentation and the frequency of systemic B symptoms, while in HIV-uninfected patients HD typically involves contiguous lymph node groups, and dissemination and infiltration of extranodal sites are late occurrences. All case reports and case series describe a particular natural history and histologic distribution of HD in infected persons that are different from those of HD in HIV-uninfected persons.[23]

The optimal treatment for HIV-related HD is controversial. Because most patients have advanced disease, the most commonly used protocols have included chemotherapy regimens used in the general population, such as MOPP, ABVD, and MOPP/ABVD. However, the complete remission rate in the HIV setting is far below the usual percentage observed in immunocompetent patients, the tolerance to chemotherapy is poor, and reduction of doses or delay of chemotherapy are often needed, resulting in a median overall survival of approximately 1.5 years.[24]

Errante et al[25] reported the results of a prospective trial with epirubicin, bleomycin, vinblastine and prednisone (EBVP) chemotherapy in combination with antiretroviral therapy and primary use of granulocyte colony-stimulating factor (G-CSF) in 35 previously untreated patients with HD and HIV infection. A complete remission rate of 74% was observed, and 10 out of 26 patients (38%) who achieved a complete remission relapsed. Twenty-three patients died of HD progression alone or in association with opportunistic infections. The median survival was 16 months, with a survival rate of 32% and a disease-free survival rate of 53% at 36 months. The authors concluded that the use of the EBVP regimen and antiretroviral treatment is feasible in the HIV setting, and, although the complete remission rate obtained was satisfactory, the relapse rate was high and the overall survival remains poor.

Currently, many clinicians believe that HD outcome in HIV patients may be improved by the optimal combination of antineoplastic and antiretroviral treatment, and the availability of HAART might also improve the control of the underlying HIV infection during chemotherapy. The inclusion of growth factors in the treatment of these patients might allow the administration of higher-dose-intensity chemotherapy as well as the prolonged use of antiretroviral drugs, and can be translated into an improvement of the overall survival.

POSSIBLE DEVELOPMENTS

In the last few years, improvements in our knowledge of the molecular pathogenesis and clinical management of AIDS-NHL has occurred. In fact, recent data on the molecular pathogenesis of systemic AIDS-NHL has led to the identification of new entities and of distinct and specific genetic pathways selectively associated with different types of AIDS-NHL. The dramatic changes seen in the incidence of opportunistic infections, and consequently in life expectancy, since the advent of HAART have encouraged more aggressive treatment of systemic AIDS-NHL. For example, high-dose chemotherapy with peripheral stem cell rescue could be tested, at least in low-risk patients with systemic AIDS-NHL, taking into consideration the adverse prognostic factors present in these patients.

Moreover, some interesting data on the use of monoclonal antibodies for the treatment of NHL in the general population have been published. In particular, rituximab, a chimeric murine/human monoclonal antibody that targets the CD20 antigen expressed on normal B cells and on more than 95% of B-cell NHL, was initially tested in the setting of low-grade lymphomas. Similar trials are also ongoing in high-grade AIDS-NHL.

In AIDS-HD, aggressive chemotherapy regimens such as Stanford V or high-dose chemotherapy with peripheral stem cell rescue should be tested, taking into consideration the good results obtained in HIV-negative patients with the same unfavorable prognostic factors that are present in AIDS-HD.

Finally, new clinical pathological subtypes are likely to emerge among both AIDS-NHL and AIDS-HD as new molecular, virologic, and clinical findings, with possible distinct evolution and response to therapy.

ACKNOWLEDGMENTS

This work was supported by ISS and AIRC grants. The authors want to thank Daniela Furlan for her expert assistance in the preparation of the manuscript.

REFERENCES

1. Tulpule A, Levine A, AIDS-related lymphoma. *Blood Rev* 1999; **13**: 147–50.

2. Grulich AE, AIDS-associated non-Hodgkin's lymphoma in the era of highly active antiretroviral therapy. *J Acq Immun Def Synd* 1999; **21**: S27–30.

3. Franceschi S, Dal Maso L, La Vecchia C, Advances in the epidemiology of HIV-associated non-Hodgkin's lymphoma and other lymphoid neoplasms. *Int J Cancer* 1999; **83**: 481–5.

4. Pezzotti P, Dal Maso L, Serraino D et al, Has the spectrum of AIDS-defining illnesses been changing since the introduction of new treatments and combination of treatments? *J Acq Immun Def Synd* 1999; **20**: 515–16.

5. Rabkin CS, Testa MA, Huang J et al, Kaposi's sarcoma and non-Hodgkin's lymphoma incidence trends in AIDS Clinical Trial Group Study participants. *J Acq Immun Def Synd* 1999; **21**: S31–3.

6. Ledergerber B, Telenti A, Egger M, for the Swiss HIV Cohort Study, Risk of HIV-related Kaposi's sarcoma and non-Hodgkin's lymphoma with potent antiretroviral therapy: prospective cohort study. *BMJ* 1999; **319**: 23–4.

7. Baiocchi RA, Caligiuri MA, Cytokines in the evolution and treatment of AIDS-lymphoma. *Curr Opin Oncol* 1999; **11**: 516–21.

8. Stylianou E, Aukrust P, Dvale D et al, IL-10 in HIV infection: increasing serum

IL-10 levels with disease progression-down-regulatory effect of potent antiretroviral therapy. *Clin Exp Immunol* 1999; **116**: 115–20.

9. Drexler HG, Meyer C, Gaidano G et al, Constitutive cytokine production by primary effusion (body cavity-based) lymphoma-derived cell lines. *Leukemia* 1999; **13**: 634–40.

10. Crabb Breen E, van der Meijden M, Cumberland W et al, The development of AIDS-associated Burkitt's/small non-cleaved cell lymphoma is preceded by elevated serum levels of interleukin 6. *Clin Immunol* 1999; **93**: 114–23.

11. Rabkin CS, Yang Q, Goedert JJ et al, Chemokine and chemokine receptor gene variants and risk of non-Hodgkin's lymphoma in human immunodeficiency virus-1-infected individuals. *Blood* 1999; **93**: 1838–42.

12. Dean M, Jacobson LP, McFarlane G et al, Reduced risk of AIDS lymphoma in individuals heterozygous for the *CCR5-Δ32* mutation. *Cancer Res* 1999; **59**: 3561–4.

13. Komano J, Maruo S, Kurozumi K et al, Oncogenic role of Epstein–Barr virus-encoded RNAs in Burkitt's lymphoma cell line Akata. *J Virol* 1999; **73**: 9827–31.

14. Schroeder JR, Saah AJ, Hoover DR et al, Serum soluble CD23 level correlates with subsequent development of AIDS-related non-Hodgkin's lymphoma. *Cancer Epidemiol Biomark* 1999; **8**: 979–84.

15. Schroeder JR, Saah AJ, Ambinder RF et al, Serum sCD23 level in patients with AIDS-related non-Hodgkin's lymphoma is associated with absence of Epstein–Barr virus in tumor tissue. *Clin Immunol* 1999; **93**: 239–44.

16. Chirivi RGS, Taraboletti G, Bani MR et al, Human immunodeficiency virus-1 (HIV-1)-tat protein promotes migration of acquired immunodeficiency syndrome-related lymphoma cells and enhances their adhesion to endothelial cells. *Blood* 1999; **94**: 1747–54.

17. Spina M, Vaccher E, Carbone A et al, Neoplastic complications of HIV infection. *Ann Oncol* 1999; **10**: 1271–86.

18. Antinori A, De Rossi G, Ammassari A et al, Value of combined approach with thallium-201 single-photon emission computed tomography and Epstein–Barr virus DNA polymerase chain reaction in CSF for the diagnosis of AIDS-related primary CNS lymphoma. *J Clin Oncol* 1999; **17**: 554–60.

19. Rossi G, Donisi A, Casari S et al, The International Prognostic Index can be used as a guide to treatment decisions regarding patients with human immunodeficiency virus-related systemic non-Hodgkin lymphoma. *Cancer* 1999; **86**: 2391–7.

20. Evison J, Jost J, Ledergerber B et al, HIV-associated non-Hodgkin's lymphoma: highly active antiretroviral therapy improves remission rate of chemotherapy. *AIDS* 1999; **13**: 732–4.

21. Campbell P, Iland H, Gibson J et al, Syngeneic stem cell transplantation for HIV-related lymphoma. *Br J Haematol* 1999; **105**: 795–8.

22. Carbone A, Gloghini A, Larocca LM et al, Human immunodeficiency virus-associated Hodgkin's disease derives from post-germinal center B cells. *Blood* 1999; **93**: 2319–26.

23. Tirelli U, Carbone A, Straus DJ, HIV-related Hodgkin's disease. In: *Hodgkin's Disease* (Mauch PM, Armitage JO, Diehl V et al, eds). Philadelphia: Lippincott Williams & Wilkins, 1999: 701–11.

24. Spina M, Sandri S, Tirelli U, Hodgkin's disease in HIV-infected individuals. *Curr Opin Oncol* 1999; **11**: 522–6.

25. Errante D, Gabarre J, Ridolfo AL et al, Hodgkin's disease in 35 patients with HIV infection: an experience with epirubicin, bleomycin, vinblastine and prednisone chemotherapy in combination with antiretroviral therapy and primary use of G-CSF. *Ann Oncol* 1999; **10**: 189–95.

10
Chronic lymphocytic leukemia

Emilio Montserrat

INTRODUCTION

Chronic lymphocytic leukemia (CLL), the most frequent form of leukemia in Western countries, is due to the accumulation of neoplastic B lymphocytes. The disease predominates in the elderly and has a variable clinical course. Important advances have been made over the last few years in the biology, natural history, and treatment of this form of leukemia.

This chapter summarizes the progress made in CLL during 1999. For a general framework of CLL, the reader may be interested in some of the reviews published in 1999.[1–6] In addition, important updated information can be found in the proceedings of the VIII Meeting of the International Workshop on CLL held in Paris this year.[7,8]

EPIDEMIOLOGY

The variability in the incidence of CLL according to race is well known. Thus, whereas in western countries, CLL accounts for about 20–40% of all leukemias, in Asian populations, it constitutes only 3–5% of the total number of cases. Interestingly, in Asians who have emigrated to the USA, the incidence of CLL remains low. CLL has also been found to be more frequent in Jews originating from Eastern Europe than in Sephardim. A recent study indicating that CLL is not frequent in Mexico (6.6% of the adult cases of leukemia) and that it is particularly rare in Mexican mestizos[9] has added another piece to this puzzle. All these differences most likely reflect genuine racial differences in CLL predisposition, although, in some cases, under- and misdiagnoses or variability in access to medical care might also account for part of the differences.

In one registry study,[10] out of 108 396 cases of leukemia, CLL comprised 22.6%. The median age of the patients at diagnosis was close to 70, and about 20% of them were 60 or older. The five-year and ten-year overall survival rates were 48.2% and 22.5%, respectively. The relative survival rate (observed survival divided by expected survival for a control population) was 66.4% at five years from diagnosis. When broken down by age, relative survival was shortened in all age groups, including the elderly. This study is a reminder that – in contrast to the view still held by some physicians – CLL is not a 'benign' disease.

Familial aggregation is not rare in CLL. The risk of leukemia in people with one or more first-degree relatives with CLL has been estimated as two- to sevenfold greater than for individuals without relatives with the disease. The mechanisms underlying this fact are unknown. An interesting observation is the so-called 'anticipation phenomenon', whereby, in younger members of the affected family, CLL presents, on average, 20 years earlier than in the older members.[11] The potential relationship between familial CLL and genetic alterations is discussed below.

DIAGNOSIS

The WHO classification considers CLL as the leukemic counterpart of small lymphocytic lymphoma, clearly separate from prolymphocytic leukemia. The presence of a monoclonal gammopathy in serum or plasmacytoid features in the leukemic cells are accepted as disease variants.[12]

The hallmark for the diagnosis is the presence in peripheral blood of a monoclonal population of small, mature-appearing B lymphocytes with a characteristic immunophenotype (surface membrane immunoglobulin (SmIg)-weak, $CD5^+$, $CD23^+$, $CD22^{weak}$, $CD79b^{- or weak}$, $FCM7^-$).

Although most CLL cases have a characteristic morphology, there are patients displaying atypical features. In such cases, a relatively simple set of cell-surface markers is useful for diagnosis. Typical CLL cases are $SmIg^{weak}$, $CD5^+$, $CD22^{weak}$, $FCM7^-$, $CD23^+$. By giving one point to each one of these markers, a diagnostic scoring system can be designed. Whereas most cases of CLL score 4 or 5, the majority of other B-cell disorders that mimic CLL score 0, 1, or 2. CD79b behaves similarly to CD22.[13]

$CD5^-$ B-cell lymphoproliferative disorders are rarely classifiable as CLL. In a large study, 41 of 192 B-cell lymphoproliferative disorders (21%) were found to be $CD5^-$. Upon careful analysis, however, only three $CD5^-$ cases (7%) were classified as CLL, but with atypical features, including a debatable case of Richter's syndrome.[14] In another similar study, it was stressed that $CD5^-$ 'CLL' cases may correspond, in many instances, to mantle-cell lymphomas in leukemic phase.[15]

The message from these studies is that the diagnosis of atypical CLL should not be accepted without carefully discarding other lymphoproliferative disorders. In this regard, not only the immunophenotype of the cells, but also cytogenetic and molecular findings can be of help (reviewed by Criel et al[16] and Pangalis et al[13]).

GENETIC ABNORMALITIES

The sensitivity with which chromosome aberrations are detected in CLL has been dramatically improved by the introduction of techniques that allow the analysis of interphase cells, such as fluorescence in situ hybridization (FISH). Chromosomal aberrations can thus be detected in more than 80% CLL cases. The most frequent aberrations are deletions of the long arm of chromosome 13, which occur in more than half of all cases. This is followed by deletion of 11q (about 20% of cases), trisomy 12 (about 15%), deletion of 17p (about 10%), and deletion of 6q (about 5%).[17,18] The search for correlates between cytogenetic abnormalities and clinical features has continued. It is well documented, for example, that trisomy 12 is associated with both atypical morphology and immunophenotype (reviewed by Criel et al[16]). In addition, deletions of 11q are observed in relatively young individuals, with bulky disease resistant to therapy; this abnormality has found to be associated with reduced expression of a number of adhesion molecules.[19] Deletions of 17p involve *p53*, and are associated with progressive disease and resistance to treatment. Finally, deletions of 6q21 are found in 7% of patients, and identify a subgroup of patients with larger tumor mass but no inferior outcome.[20]

No gene has yet been found to be consistently involved in the pathogenesis of CLL. Thus, none of the proto-oncogenes associated with other mature B-cell malignancies, such as *CCND1* (encoding cyclin D1), *BCL2*, *BCL6*, *PAX5*, and c-*MYC*, are primarily altered in this disease.

The most likely region for a gene related to CLL is 13q14.3. This region is telomeric to the retinoblastoma gene *RB1* and centromeric to a region that includes the D13S25 marker. The race to identify the gene (or genes) in this region involved in CLL has continued – unfortunately with no more than negative results. The *Leu1* and *Leu2* genes, for example, have been excluded as tumor suppressor genes involved in CLL.[21]

Among the genes most widely studied is the *ATM* gene, which is localized in chromosomal region 11q22.3–q23.1. In CLL, *ATM* mutations have been found in subsets of cases with 11q deletions and a poor prognosis.[22–24]

On the other hand, one study of the relationship between *ATM* abnormalities and familial CLL has given negative results.[25] In an analysis of the Ig V gene in familial cases of CLL, it was found that Ig V-gene segment utilization was not random, with preferential involvement of the 3–23 gene segment, as well as a high degree of somatic mutations. These findings were interpreted as indicating that familial CLL cases may preferentially derive from B-cell progenitors that have responded to antigens.[26]

CLL has long been considered a homogeneous disease of naive CD5$^+$ B cells, pre-germinal cells not exposed to antigenic stimulation. In 1999, two different groups reported an important breakthrough in CLL.[27,28] These groups have clearly shown that the mutational status of the Ig V gene correlates with different disease subsets. Thus, those patients with unmutated Ig V gene ('naive' or 'pre-germinal' CLL) have a poorer prognosis than those displaying a mutated

Ig V gene ('memory' or 'post-germinal' CLL). Hamblin et al[27] analyzed the Ig V-gene sequences of 84 patients with CLL, and demonstrated two patterns: 38 (45%) showed over 98% sequence homology with germline Ig V gene, whereas 46 (55%) showed evidence of somatic mutation. Since somatic mutation takes place in the germinal center, CLL can be either a tumor of naive, pre-germinal-centre B cells or a tumor of post-germinal-center, memory B cells. CLL deriving from naive cells is more likely to have an advanced stage ($p = 0.0009$), progressive disease ($p < 0.0001$), atypical morphology ($p = 0.0001$), trisomy 12 as a single chromosomal abnormality ($p = 0.0019$), and a shorter survival irrespective of stage. Patients with stage A CLL have a median survival of 8 years if the CLL derives from naive B cells and 25 years if it derives from memory B cells ($p = 0.0008$).[27]

Unfortunately, most laboratories are currently unable to isolate and characterize Ig V-gene sequences. However, the finding by Damle et al[28] that CD38 status correlates with Ig V-gene mutations (i.e., $CD38^+ \geqslant 30\%$ with unmutated Ig V genes; $CD38^+ < 30\%$ with mutated Ig V genes) may have important practical consequences). Nevertheless, the value of CD38 as a surrogate of the Ig V-gene mutational status is disputed and would require confirmation.

APOPTOSIS AND MICROENVIRONMENT

Although most CLL B lymphocytes are in the G_0 phase of the cell cycle, these cells undergo spontaneous programmed cell death by apoptosis when cultivated in vitro. This indicates that the microenvironment plays a key role in preventing apoptosis. The mechanisms accounting for this are complex. Adhesion of CLL cells to stromal cells, which is basically mediated by β_1- and β_2-integrins, prevents apoptosis (reviewed by Angelopoulou et al[29] and by Lagneaux et al[30]). On the other hand, fibronectin has been shown to upregulate the BCL2/BAX ratio in in vitro experiments.[31]

Another important feature in CLL is the tendency of the neoplastic lymphocytes to accumulate in bone marrow and lymphoid tissues. CLL B lymphocytes express functional CXCR4 receptors for the chemokine stromal cell-derived factor 1 (SDF-1), as well as CXCR3. These receptors mediate the adherence of the leukemic cells to marrow stromal cells.[32–34] CLL cells have also been shown to adhere to hyaluronan, becoming motile when stimulated with interleukin (IL)-8. Blocking antibodies showed that this motility is mediated by the receptor for hyaluronan-mediated motility.[35] On the other hand, downregulation of L-selectin and CD23 has been related to impaired transendothelial migration of lymphocytes in CLL.[36] These, and many other similar studies, indicate the importance of microenvironment and cell-to-cell signaling in the pathogenesis of CLL (reviewed by Caligaris-Cappio and Hamblin[1]).

Finally, abnormalities in the B-cell receptor (BCR) have received much attention. The BCR of the mature B cell is a multimeric complex that is formed by the SmIg homodimer and the non-covalently bound heterodimer Igα/Igβ

(CD79a/CD79b). The expression of the extracellular domain of CD79b is absent or weak, leading to defective BCR-mediated signal transduction. This has been related to abnormalities in the CD79b gene.[37,38]

PROGNOSIS

In recent series, the median survival of patients with CLL is close to 10 years. Clinical stages, degree of bone marrow infiltration, and doubling time are the most useful parameters for predicting survival. Cytogenetic abnormalities are also very important prognostic factors.[17,18,39,40] Thus, patients with del(13q) as a single abnormality have an excellent prognosis (median survival 133 months), whereas those with del(11q) or del(17p) have poor survival (median survival 79 and 32 months, respectively).[18]

Efforts have been made to refine the concept of *smoldering CLL*. Hallek et al[41] showed that serum levels of thymidine kinase (>7.1 U/l), presence of lymphadenopathy, and white cell count higher than 75 000/µl are independent prognostic factors in early (Binet stage A) disease. In another study, serum levels of vascular endothelial growth factor (VEGF) predicted the risk of disease progression in early CLL.[42] Future studies should be aimed at determining parameters associated to indolent disease regardless of the clinical stage, the reason being that smoldering disease is not limited to early-stage disease but can be observed in all disease stages.

Molica et al[43] analyzed the natural history of 204 patients from a single institution in early (Binet A) stage. The risk of disease progression was 32.8% at five years and 49.6% at ten years from diagnosis. Disease progression had a clearly negative influence on survival. Of note, however, survival of patients who progressed was similar to that of patients in the same stage at diagnosis. These results support the notion that only patients with symptomatic or progressive disease should be treated.

Another study focused on the outcome of a large series of younger patients.[44] As previously reported by others, younger and older patients displayed similar features at diagnosis, except for a higher male-to-female ratio in younger patients (2.85 versus 1.29; $p < 0.0001$). Both groups showed a high incidence of second cancers (8.3% versus 10.7%), whereas the occurrence of Richter syndrome was significantly higher in younger patients (5.9% versus 1.2%; $p < 0.00001$). In the multivariate analysis, lymphocyte doubling time and other disease progression parameters were the only significant features predicting survival. Such studies help in identifying younger patients in whom experimental treatments are warranted.

The prognostic implications of mutations of the Ig *V* gene[27,28] have been discussed above under 'Genetic abnormalities'.

TREATMENT

Treatment of CLL should be planned according to the individual risk of each patient.[45] Whereas important progress has been made regarding *what* type of patients require therapy and *when* treatment should be initiated, *how* to treat CLL – that is, the most appropriate treatment in each situation – is still unclear. A number of interesting new treatments, such as monoclonal antibodies (e.g., Campath-1H, rituximab), cytotoxic agents (bryostatin, depsipeptide, flavopiridol, UCN-01), and vaccines, are under investigation. Given their experimental nature, these treatments are not covered in this chapter; however, the interested reader may refer to specific papers[46–49] and to a comprehensive review.[50]

In the chemotherapy field, the results of a large meta-analysis have been published.[51] Immediate treatment with chlorambucil alone or chlorambucil plus prednisone/prednisolone was compared with deferred therapy on the basis of the analysis of six trials, including 2048 patients. The 10-year survival rate was slightly worse, although not statistically significant, with immediate chemotherapy (44% versus 47%). In addition, there were another 2022 patients in ten trials of combination chemotherapy versus chlorambucil with or without prednisone/prednisolone. Again, no differences were observed, the five-year survival rate being 48% in both cases.

The notion that patients with early disease should not be treated unless they progress is now one of the paradigms in CLL. It should be noted, however, that chlorambucil was the drug employed in all the trials on which this idea is based. The correct interpretation is not, therefore, that *treatment* is not useful in early-stage CLL but rather that *chlorambucil* does not improve the outcome of such patients. This raises the question of whether the outcome of these patients, particularly those with active, non-smoldering disease, could be improved by new and more effective treatments – an issue now being investigated.

Purine analogues are the most effective agents in CLL, although unfortunately the higher response rate achieved with these drugs does not translate into a longer survival. Reports dealing with purine analogues in the treatment of CLL, as well as complications related to these drugs, have been published.[52–54]

From a practical point of view, the availability of fludarabine in oral form will greatly facilitate the treatment of patients with CLL.[55] In a multicenter, uncontrolled, open-label study, oral fludarabine phosphate was administered at a dose of 40 mg/m²/day for 5 days, every 4 weeks, for 6–8 cycles, to 78 patients with symptomatic CLL. The overall response rate was 51.3% (17.9% complete and 33.3% partial). In general, the efficacy of oral fludarabine phosphate seems to be comparable to that observed with the intravenous formulation.[56]

One of the challenges in CLL is to increase the complete response rate, particularly if achieving complete response is deemed necessary in the treatment strategy, such as when an autologous transplant is planned. Bellosillo et al[57] have demonstrated the synergism of fludarabine with cyclophosphamide and mitoxantrone in in vitro studies, giving support to trials that investigate these, and other, agents in combination.[57–61]

About one-third of CLL patients are under the age of 60. In this group of patients, the aim of treatment cannot merely be one of symptom palliation. Young patients with high-risk disease are good candidates for experimental trials. In this context, the number of transplants in CLL is dramatically increasing.[62]

In the autologous transplantation setting, transplant-related mortality is usually less than 10%, and the status of the disease at the time of transplantation is the most important factor for survival. As far as disease-free survival is concerned, the status of the disease before transplantation, along with the number of previous lines of treatment, is again the most important prognostic factor. Of note, the survival plots do now show a plateau, and there is a constant pattern of relapses (about 50% at four years post transplant), suggesting that autologous transplants do not cure CLL. On the other hand, the absence of minimal residual disease after transplantation correlates with a longer disease-free interval[63–65] (reviewed by Popplewell and Forman[66]).

Allogeneic transplants result in a transplant-related mortality ranging from 25% to 50%. In contrast to autologous transplants, however, in most series, there is a survival plateau of about 40%; this is probably due, at least in part, to a graft-versus-CLL effect. As with autologous transplants, the absence of minimal residual disease after transplantation is associated with a longer disease-free interval (again reviewed by Popplewell and Forman[66]).

The use of non-myeloablative regimens in allogeneic transplants is appealing because they could contribute to decreasing the transplant-related-mortality and to increasing the age limit of transplantable patients (reviewed by Champlin et al[67]).

FUTURE TRENDS

Over the last 10 years, important progress has been made in CLL. Future studies should continue to unfold the biological and clinical heterogeneity of this form of leukemia. Prognostic models based on clinical and biological features should be developed. Such efforts should throw new light on our understanding of CLL. Ultimately, this should lead to the development not only of risk-adapted (i.e., based on prognostic factors) but also of disease-adapted (i.e., based on biological diversity) treatment strategies. Purine analogues in combination with other drugs, therapies based on the combined use of chemotherapy and biological agents (e.g, monoclonal antibodies), hematopoietic stem cell transplants, and immunological manipulation should continue to be investigated. Fortunately, after many decades of stagnation, the possibility of not only improving the outcome of most patients with CLL but also curing some of them is on the horizon.

REFERENCES

1. Caligaris-Cappio F, Hamblin TJ, B-cell chronic lymphocytic leukemia: a bird of a different feather. *J Clin Oncol* 1999; 17: 399–408.

2. Kalil N, Cheson BD, Chronic lymphocytic leukemia. *Oncologist* 1999; 4: 352–69.

3. Keating MJ (Chair), Caligaris-Cappio F, Bullrich F et al, Translational research in chronic lymphocytic leukemia. In: *Hematology 1999 – American Society of Hematology Education Program Book*: 249–69.

4. Oscier D, Chronic lymphocytic leukemia. *Br J Haematol* 1999; 105(Suppl 1): 1–3.

5. Rai KR (Chair), Byrd JC, Foa R (Speakers), Chronic lymphocytic leukemia. In: *Am Soc Clin Oncol 1999 Educational Book*: 164–83.

6. Wierda WG, Kipps TJ, Chronic lymphocytic leukemia. *Curr Opin Hematol* 1999; 6: 253–61.

7. Meeting Report: VIII International Workshop on CLL. *Leuk Lymphoma Updates* 1999; 2: 3–21.

8. International Workshop on CLL (IWCLL): Report of the VIII International Workshop. *Hematol Cell Ther* 2000; 42: 1–116.

9. Ruiz-Argüelles GJ, Velazquez BM, Apreza-Molñina MG et al, Chronic lymphocytic leukemia is infrequent in Mexican mestizos. *Int J Hematol* 1999; 69: 253–5.

10. Diehl LF, Karnell LH, Menck HR, The national cancer data base on age, gender, treatment, and outcomes of patients with chronic lymphocytic leukemia. *Cancer* 1999; 86: 2684–92.

11. Goldin LR, Sgambati M, Marti GE et al, Anticipation in familial chronic lymphocytic leukemia. *Am J Hum Genet* 1999; 65: 265–9.

12. Harris NL, Jaffe ES, Diebold J et al, World Health Organization classification of neoplastic diseases of the hematopoietic and lymphoid tissues: report of the Clinical Advisory Committee Meeting – Airlie House, Virginia, November 1997. *J Clin Oncol* 1999; 17: 3835–49.

13. Pangalis GA, Angelopoulou MK, Vassilakopoulos TP et al, B-chronic lymphocytic leukemia, small lymphocytic leukemia, and lymphoplasmacytic lymphoma, including Waldenström's macroglobulinemia: a clinical, morphologic, and biologic spectrum of similar disorders. *Semin Hematol* 1999; 36: 104–14.

14. Huang JC, Finn WG, Goolsby CL et al, CD5⁻ small B-cell leukemias are rarely classifiable as chronic lymphocytic leukemia. *Am J Clin Pathol* 1999; 111: 123–30.

15. Shapiro JL, Miller ML, Pohlman B et al, CD5⁻ B-cell lymphoproliferative disorders presenting in blood and bone marrow. A clinicopathologic study of 40 patients. *Am J Clin Pathol* 1999; 111: 477–87.

16. Criel A, Michaux L, De Wolf-Peeters C, The concept of typical and atypical chronic lymphocytic leukaemia. *Leuk Lymphoma* 1999; 33: 33–45.

17. Döhner D, Stilgenbauer S, Döhner K et al, Chromosome aberrations in B-cell chronic lymphocytic leukemia: reassessment based on molecular cytogenetic analysis. *J Mol Med* 1999; 7: 266–81.

18. Stilgenbauer S, Leupolt E, Kröbe A et al, Molecular cytogenetic analysis of B-CLL: incidence and prognostic significance of the most frequent chromosome aberrations. *Blood* 1999; 94(Suppl 1):543.

19. Sembries S, Pahl H, Stilgenbauer S et al, Reduced expression of adhesion molecules and cell signaling receptors by chronic lymphocytic leukemia cells with 11q deletions. *Blood* 1999; 93: 624–31.

20. Stilgenbauer S, Bullinger L, Benner A et al, Incidence and clinical significance of 6q deletions in B cell chronic lymphocytic leukemia. *Leukemia* 1999; 13: 1313–34.

21. Rondeau G, Moreau I, Bézieau S et al, Exclusion of Leu1 and Leu2 genes as tumor suppressor genes in 13q14.3-deleted B-CLL. *Leukemia* 1999; **13**: 1630–2.

22. Bullrich F, Rasio D, Kitada S et al, ATM mutations in B-cell chronic lymphocytic leukemia. *Cancer Res* 1999; **59**: 24–7.

23. Schaffner C, Stilgenbauer S, Rappold GA et al, Somatic ATM mutations indicate a pathogenic role of ATM in B-cell chronic lymphocytic leukemia. *Blood* 1999; **94**: 748–53.

24. Stankovic T, Weber P, Stewart G et al, Inactivation of ataxia telangiectasia mutated gene in B-cell chronic lymphocytic leukaemia. *Lancet* 1999; **353**: 26–9.

25. Bevan S, Catovsky D, Marossy A et al, Linkage analysis for ATM in familial B cell chronic lymphocytic leukemia. *Leukemia* 1999; **13**: 1497–500.

26. Pritsch O, Troussard X, Magnac C et al, V_H gene usage by family members affected with chronic lymphocytic leukaemia. *Br J Haematol* 1999; **107**: 616–24.

27. Hamblin TJ, Davis Z, Gardiner A et al, Unmutated immunoglobulin V_H genes are associated with a more aggressive form of chronic lymphocytic leukemia. *Blood* 1999; **94**: 1848–54.

28. Damle RN, Wasil T, Fais F et al, Ig V gene mutation status and CD38 expression as novel prognostic indicators in chronic lymphocytic leukemia. *Blood* 1999; **94**: 1840–7.

29. Angelopoulou MK, Kontopidou FN, Pangalis GA, Adhesion molecules in B-chronic lymphoproliferative disorders. *Semin Hematol* 1999; **36**: 178–97.

30. Lagneaux L, Delforge A, de Bruyn C et al, Adhesion to bone marrow stroma inhibits apoptosis of chronic lymphocytic leukemia cells. *Leuk Lymphoma* 1999; **35**: 445–53.

31. de La Fuente MT, Casanova B, García-Gila M et al, Fibronectin interaction with alpha4beta1 integrin prevents apoptosis in B cell chronic lymphocytic leukemia: correlation with Bcl-2 and Bax. *Leukemia* 1999; **13**: 266–74.

32. Burger JA, Burger M, Kipps TJ, Chronic lymphocytic leukemia B cells express functional CXCR4 chemokine receptors that mediate spontaneous migration beneath bone marrow stromal cells. *Blood* 1999; **94**: 3658–67.

33. Möhle R, Failenschmid C, Bautz F, Kantz L, Overexpression of the chemokine receptor CXCR4 in B cell chronic lymphocytic leukemia is associated with increased functional response to stromal cell-derived factor-1 (SDF-1). *Leukemia* 1999; **13**: 1954–9.

34. Trentin L, Agostini C, Facco M et al, The chemokine receptor CXCR3 is expressed on malignant B cells and mediates chemotaxis. *J Clin Invest* 1999; **104**: 115–21.

35. Till J, Zuzel M, Cawley JC, The role of hyaluronan and interleukin 8 in the migration of chronic lymphocytic leukemia cells within lymphoreticular tissues. *Cancer Res* 1999; **59**: 4419–26.

36. Chen JR, Gu BJ, Dao LP et al, Transendothelial migration of lymphocytes in chronic lymphocytic leukaemia is impaired and involved down-regulation of both L-selectin and CD23. *Br J Haematol* 1999; **105**: 181–9.

37. Alfarano A, Indraccolo S, Circosta P et al, An alternative spliced form of CD79b gene may account for altered B-cell receptor expression in B-chronic lymphocytic leukemia. *Blood* 1999; **93**: 2327–35

38. Thompson AA, Do HN, Saxon A, Wall R, Widespread B29 (CD79b) gene defects and loss of expression in chronic lymphocytic leukemia. *Leuk Lymphoma* 1999; **32**: 561–9.

39. Hogan WJ, Tefferi, Borell TJ et al, Prognostic relevance of monosomy at the 13q14 locus detected by fluorescence in situ hybridization in B-cell chronic lymphocytic leukemia. *Cancer Genet Cytogenet* 1999; **110**: 77–81.

40. Starostik P, O'Brien S, Chung CY et al, The prognostic significance of 13q14 deletions in chronic lymphocytic leukemia. *Leuk Res* 1999; **23**: 795–801.

41. Hallek M, Langenmayer I, Nerl C et

al, Elevated serum thymidine kinase levels identify a subgroup at high risk of disease progression in early, nonsmoldering chronic lymphocytic leukemia. *Blood* 1999; **93**: 1732–7.

42. Molica S, Vitelli G, Levato D et al, Increased serum levels of vascular endothelial growth factor predict risk of progression in early B-cell chronic lymphocytic leukaemia. *Br J Haematol* 1999; **107**: 605–10.

43. Molica S, Levato D, Dattilo A, Natural history of early chronic lymphocytic leukemia. A single institution study with emphasis on the impact of disease progression on overall survival. *Haematologica* 1999; **84**: 1094–9.

44. Mauro FR, Foa R, Gianarelli D et al, Clinical characteristics and outcome of young chronic lymphocytic leukemia patients: a single institution study of 204 cases. *Blood* 1999; **94**: 448–54.

45. Wendtner CM, Schmitt B, Wilhelm M et al, Redefining the therapeutic goals in chronic lymphocytic leukemia: towards evidence-based, risk-adapted therapies. *Ann Oncol* 1999; **40**: 505–9.

46. Byrd JS, Shinn C, Ravi R et al, Depsipeptide (FR901228): a novel therapeutic agent with selective, in vitro activity against human B-cell chronic lymphocytic leukemia cells. *Blood* 1999; **94**: 1401–8.

47. Byrd JC, Waselenko JK, Maneatis TJ et al, Rituximab therapy in hematologic malignancy patients with circulating blood tumor cells: association with increased infusion-related side effects and rapid blood tumor clearance. *J Clin Oncol* 1999; **17**: 791–5.

48. Keating MJ, Byd J, Rai K et al, Multicenter study of Campath-1H in patients with chronic lymphocytic leukemia (B-CLL) refractory to fludarabine. *Blood* 1999; **94**(Suppl 1):705.

49. Winkler U, Jensen M, Manzke O et al, Cytokine-release syndrome in patients with B-cell chronic lymphocytic leukemia and high lymphocyte counts after treatment with anti-CD20 monoclonal antibody (rituximab, IDEC-C2B8). *Blood* 1999; **94**: 2217–24.

50. Cheson BD (Guest Ed), Future strategies toward the cure of indolent B-cell malignancies. *Semin Hematol* 1999; **36**(Suppl 5): 1–33.

51. CLL Trialists's Collaborative Group, Chemotherapeutic options in chronic lymphocytic leukemia: a meta-analysis of the randomized trials. *J Natl Cancer Inst* 1999; **91**: 861–8.

52. Cheson BD, Vena DA, Barrett J, Freidlin B, Second malignancies as a consequence of nucleoside analog therapy for chronic lymphocytic leukemia. *J Clin Oncol* 1999; **17**: 2454–60.

53. Robak T, Blasinska-Morawiec M, Blonski JZ, Dmoszynska A, 2-Chlorodeoxyadenosine (cladribine) in the treatment of elderly patients with B-cell chronic lymphocytic leukemia. *Leuk Lymphoma* 1999; **34**: 151–7.

54. Robak T, Blonski JZ, Urbanska-Rys H et al, 2-Chlorodeoxyadenosine (cladribine) in the treatment of patients with chronic lymphocytic leukemia 55 years old and younger. *Br J Haematol* 1999; **13**: 518–23.

55. Foran JM, Oscier D, Orchad J et al, Pharmacokinetic study of single doses of oral fludarabine phosphate in patients with 'low-grade' non-Hodgkin's lymphoma and B-cell chronic lymphocytic leukemia. *J Clin Oncol* 1999; **17**: 1574–9.

56. Boogaerts M, Van Hoff A, Catovsky D et al, treatment of alkylator resistant chronic lymphocytic leukemia with oral fludarabine phosphate. *Blood* 1999; **94**(Suppl 1): 704.

57. Bellosillo B, Villamor N, Colomer D et al, In vitro evaluation of fludarabine in combination with cyclophosphamide and/or mitoxantrone in B-cell chronic lymphocytic leukemia. *Blood* 1999; **94**: 2836–43.

58. Frewin R, Turner D, Tighe M et al, Combination therapy with fludarabine and cyclophosphamide as salvage treatment in lymphoproliferative disorders. *Br J Haematol* 1999; **104**: 612–13.

59. Giles FJ, O'Brien SM, Santini V et al, Sequential cis-platinum and fludarabine with or without arabinosyl cytosine in

patients failing prior fludarabine therapy for chronic lymphocytic leukemia: a phase II study. *Leuk Lymphoma* 1999; **36**: 57–65.

60. Rummel MJ, Kafer G, Pfreundschuh M et al, Fludarabine and epirubicin in the treatment of chronic lymphocytic leukaemia: a German multicenter phase II study. *Ann Oncol* 1999; **10**: 183–8.

61. Tosi P, Pellacani A, Zinzani PL et al, In vitro study of the combination gemcitabine + fludarabine on freshly isolated chronic lymphocytic leukemia cells. *Haematologica* 1999; **84**: 794–8.

62. Gratwohl A, Passweg J, Baldomero H, Hermans J, Blood and marrow transplantation activity in Europe 1997. European Group for Blood and Marrow Transplantation (EBMT). *Bone Marrow Transplant* 1999; **24**: 231–45.

63. Montserrat E, Esteve J, Schmitz N et al, Autologous stem-cell transplantation (ASCT) for chronic lymphocytic leukemia (CLL): results in 107 patients. *Blood* 1999; **94**(Suppl 1): 397.

64. Schey SA, Ahsan G, Jones R, Dose intensification and molecular responses in patients with chronic lymphocytic leukaemia: a phase II single center study. *Bone Marrow Transplant* 1999; **24**: 989–93.

65. Waselenko JK, Flynn JM, Byrd JC, Stem-cell transplantation in chronic lymphocytic leukemia: the time for designing randomized studies has arrived. *Semin Oncol* 1999; **26**: 48–61.

66. Popplewell L, Forman SJ, Allogeneic hematopoietic stem cell transplantation for acute leukemia, chronic leukemia, and myelodysplasia. *Hematol Oncol Clin North Am* 1999; **13**: 987–1016.

67. Champlin R, Khouri I, Kornblau S et al, Allogeneic hematopoietic transplantation as adoptive immunotherapy: induction of graft-versus-malignancy as primary therapy. *Hematol Oncol Clin North Am* 1999; **13**: 1041–57.

11
Multiple myeloma

Gösta Gahrton

STATE-OF-THE-ART

Multiple myeloma is a malignant disease with a median survival of about three years when conventional chemotherapy is used. Although the etiology is unknown, several factors of importance for the pathogenesis of the disease have previously been described. Most important is the cytokine interleukin-6 (IL-6), which promotes the growth of malignant plasma cells. A number of other cytokines, adhesion molecules, and transcription factors promote or suppress IL-6 or may have effects through other mechanisms directly on the myeloma cells. Proteins of importance include, among others, BAX, BCLX$_L$, BCL2, p53, RAS, RB1, NF-κB, AP1, NFIL6, STAT1 and STAT3, and the metalloproteinases (e.g. interstitial collagenase (MMP1) and gelatinases (MMP2 and MMP9)). Much work has been done to identify interactions between these proteins and their importance for myeloma development, regression, or progression. IL-6 still appears to be the key protein in the pathogenesis of the disease.

Cytogenetics and fluoresence in situ hybridization (FISH) analysis have shown complex karyotypes, and certain aberrations, such as deletions on chromosomes 13 and 11, appear to be most important for prognosis. On the molecular level, the immunoglobulin (Ig) heavy-chain locus may be involved in 14q13 aberrations and the retinoblastoma (*RB1*) gene in 13q aberrations.

A heated debate is ongoing concerning the etiologic role of a possible Kaposi's sarcoma-associated herpesvirus/human herpesvirus 8 (KSHV/HHV8) infection of dendritic cells in the marrow. The hypothesis has been proposed that KSHV infection of these cells could promote viral IL-6 and thereby the development of multiple myeloma.

The treatment of patients has changed from conventional chemotherapy with melphalan plus prednisolone or other chemotherapeutic drug combinations to the use of high-dose treatment followed by autologous hematopoietic stem cell transplantation or in some cases allogeneic transplantation. In 1999, some advances were made in both autologous and allogeneic stem cell transplantation, and new drugs have been tried – in particular, the antiangiogenic drug thalidomide.

A search on the Internet reveals 718 references about multiple myeloma in 1999, and 364 of them concern treatment. Reference will be made to a small fraction of these, but also to some new results presented at the VIIth International Multiple Myeloma Workshop in Stockholm, in September 1999. Thus, the review in this chapter will be highly selective, and will focus on new treatment methods.

ETIOLOGY AND PATHOGENESIS

The previous claim of KSHV infection of bone marrow dendritic cells and its possible association with multiple myeloma has been strongly challenged by several groups.[1] Firstly, with one exception, antibodies could not be found by several groups who investigated multiple myeloma patients, irrespective of the methodology used. The exception was a South African study,[2] which found a seroprevalence rate of 24% in 108 myeloma patients. However, in the control material of 3293 patients with cancer other than Kaposi's sarcoma, the rate was 32%. In Kaposi's sarcoma, the rate was 83%. Thus myeloma patients could raise an antibody response to KSHV, but the rate of seroprevalence was no higher than in other cancer patients – arguing against an association. Secondly, most groups also failed to show that myeloma patients were infected by KSHV. Tarte et al[1] made a thorough investigation and claimed that four studies have failed to confirm the original observation by Rettig et al[3] that cultured stromal dendritic cells from multiple myeloma patients were infected with KSHV. Tarte et al concluded that all studies eight months after the initial publication by Rettig et al had failed to confirm a widespread infection of bone marrow stromal cells in multiple myeloma, and 14 of 15 studies showed lack of KSHV seroprevalence in myeloma, in contrast to other KSHV-related diseases. Furthermore, it was shown in one study[2] that there was no lack of capacity of myeloma patients to raise a response. However, in three studies, some amplification of the KS330 sequence related to ORF26 was confirmed from either both marrow cultures or bone marrow biopsies. Chauhan et al[4] could show that 24 out of 26 myeloma patients (92%), but only 1 out of 4 normal donors, were KSHV polymerase chain reaction (PCR)-positive, using first a PCR reaction with primers that amplify a KSHV gene sequence to yield 233 bp fragments, which were then used as templates in a subsequent nested PCR with primers that amplify a 186 bp product internal to KS330233. The KSHV PCR-positive bone marrow cells in the patients demonstrated expression of dendritic cell lineage markers (CD68, CD83, and fascin). However, lytic or latent antibodies to KSHV were not found. Thus, these studies partly confirmed the previous study by Rettig et al.[3] Additional work by Berenson and Vescio[5] also confirms their original observation. A working group was formed at the VIIth International Multiple Myeloma Workshop with the aim of finding a strategy to clarify the role of KSHV in multiple myeloma and the possible role of viral IL-6 in the etiology and pathogenesis of the disease.

Cytogenetic aberrations have been studied both in myeloma patients and in myeloma cell lines. Bergsagel et al[6] have mapped and cloned several breakpoints, and have identified genes in close proximity to the breakpoints 11q13, 16q23, and 4p16: *CCND1* (encoding cyclin D1) is 10–300 kb telomeric of 11q13, c-*MAF* is within 500 kb of 16q23, and the fibroblast growth factor receptor 3 gene (*FGFR3*) is 50–100 kb telomeric of 4p16. The breakpoints on 4p fall within the introns of a new gene, *MMSET*. All of these genes are dysregulated, and progression of myeloma is associated with the development of activating mutations in *FGFR3* or *RAS*, but not both. On the basis of these results, Bergsagel et al have proposed a multistep model of malignant transformation of multiple myeloma that is initiated by an Ig gene translocation that results in the ectopic expression of an oncogene (*CCND1*, c-*MAF*, *FGFR3/MMSET*) caused by its juxtaposition to Ig regulatory elements. There is early acquisition of chromosomal instability and subsequently activating mutations of *RAS* or *FGFR3*.

Chromosomal aberrations were found to be clinically most important. Some of them (e.g., 13q deletions combined with 11q aberrations) were associated with very poor prognosis. In multivariate analysis, these aberrations are the most important prognostic factor following autologous transplantation.[7] Monosomy of chromosome 13 has been implicated as a step in the transition from monoclonal gammopathy of undetermined significance (MGUS) to multiple myeloma.[8] Using FISH analysis, monosomy 13 was found in 31% of myeloma patients without a history of MGUS, but in 70% of those with preceeding MGUS. It was only found in 4 out of 19 MGUS patients, and only in a minor subset of the plasma cells, while in myeloma, the majority of the cells had the deletion.

TREATMENT

Conventional treatment with melphalan plus prednisolone or VAD (vincristine, doxorubicin, and dexamethasone) has not changed significantly for patients older than 65–70 years. Autologous transplantation has been the treatment of choice for most patients under 65 years of age, and for a fraction of patients allogeneic transplantation has been indicated. Recently, non-myeloablative transplantation has been tried with some success.

Autologous transplantation

Several studies in 1999 aimed at reducing the number of tumor cells in the autologous graft by positive selection of CD34$^+$ stem cells. Results are available mainly for two systems, either the Ceprate SC (CellPro Inc.) or the Isolex-3000 device (Nexell). Previous studies have shown that the tumor cell load is reduced. The studies in 1999 focused mainly on evaluation of engraftment efficacy and on comparison of engraftment with CD34-selected versus non-selected peripheral blood stem cells (PBSC). In one study[9] of 30 patients, a linear reduction in clonal myeloma cells was seen using a highly sensitive seminested PCR technique. The lowest detection limit was 1 myeloma cell/10^6 cells. Myeloma cells were still detected in 29 out of the 30 samples from the CD34-enriched fraction. The CD34-selection procedure resulted in a median 28-fold enrichment of CD34$^+$ hematopoietic precursor cells. Thus, although there was a 2.15-log reduction in the number of clonal cells (99.3%), clonal cells were still present in the graft. There is unanimous agreement that selected CD34$^+$ cells will engraft – but perhaps with a slower rate than unselected cells. In a small case-matched study,[10] the median times to neutrophils $\geqslant 0.5 \times 10^9/l$ platelet count $\geqslant 50 \times 10^9/l$ were 14 and 23 days with CD34-selected PBSC and 11 and 14 days with non-selected PBSC, which was significantly favorable. At a median follow-up of 32 months, there were no significant differences in survival or progression-free survival between the two groups.

The most important comparison was made by Vesico et al.[11] One-hundred and thirty-one multiple myeloma patients were randomized to receive either an autologous transplant with CD34-selected cells or unselected PBSC after myeloablative therapy. Tumor cell contamination in the autograft was assessed by a quantitative PCR detection assay using patient-specific, complementarity-determining region Ig gene primers before and after selection. A median 3.1-log reduction of contaminating tumor cells was achieved in the CD34-selected product using the Ceprate SC system. No significant difference in engraftment was seen in patients who received an infused dose of at least 2×10^6 CD34$^+$ cells/kg. The follow-up time and the size of the study did not make it possible to make comparison between progression-free or overall survivals.

Thus, CD34 sorting using any available cell-sorting system can reduce the tumor cell load, and in most cases can retain enough CD34$^+$ cells to obtain a safe engraftment. Also, it appears that if the number of CD34$^+$ cells transfused is more than $2 \times 10^6/l$, there may not be a significant difference in time to engraftment between CD34-sorted and non-sorted PBSC.

It is possible that the yield of CD34$^+$ cells can be improved by adding stem cell factor (SCF) to filgrastim (recombinant human granulocyte colony-stimulating factor, G-CSF). One randomized study compared stem cell factor in combination with filgrastim after chemotherapy versus filgrastim alone.[12] One-hundred and two patients with multiple myeloma were randomized to receive mobilization chemotherapy with cyclophosphamide, SCF, and filgrastim or cyclophosphamide and filgrastim alone. Patients receiving the combination had a threefold greater chance of reaching 5×10^6 CD34$^+$ cells/kg in a single leukapheresis compared with those who were mobilized with filgrastim alone. The median CD34$^+$ cell yield was 11.3×10^6/kg in the SCF group versus 4.0×10^6/kg in the filgrastim-alone group. Thus, if CD34 selection appears advantageous in future studies, the cell dose might be of great importance. Adding SCF improves the possibility of obtaining enough CD34$^+$ cells for such approaches.

Another approach to improve the results of autologous transplantation has been to perform tandem transplants. The importance of this methodology is still unclear. Barlogie et al[7] used tandem transplants between 1990 and 1995 in 231 patients who were enrolled in a so-called total-therapy program. All patients had stage III multiple myeloma. Twenty-six percent obtained a complete remission and 75% a partial remission after the first transplant, and 41% and 83%, respectively, after the second transplant. Median overall and event-free survivals were 68 and 43 months, respectively.

An EBMT (European Group for Blood and Marrow Transplantation) registry study indicates that a second transplant, whether planned or unplanned, improves survival compared with a single transplant, with no difference between planned and unplanned second transplants.[13] However, recently the Intergroupe Français du Myélome, in a randomized study, has not found any significant difference in overall or progression-free survival between single or tandem transplants at a median follow up of three years, provided that all 402 randomized patients were included in an intention-to-treat analysis. For patients with β_2-microglobulin less than 3 mg/l a significant difference, to the advantage of tandem transplantation, was found.[14] Thus, the role of tandem transplants is not yet settled, although there are indications that perhaps survival can be somewhat improved for subsets of patients. It may not be necessary to plan the second transplant soon after the first one. Most unplanned second transplants in the EBMT study were performed because of progression of the disease. This approach may be the more cost-effective.

Allogeneic transplantation

Recent updates of allogeneic transplants reported to the EBMT registry have shown dramatic improvements in recent years.[15] The overall median survival for all transplants performed during 1983–1993 was 12 months from the time of transplantation, while it was 43 months in transplants during 1994–1998. The transplant-related mortality was 40% and 20%, respectively, during these two time periods. The overall survival for transplants performed with PBSC from 1994 to 1998 was not significantly different from the overall survival with bone marrow during this time, although there was a tendency for higher transplant-related mortality with PBSC. The relapse rate was similar in all groups. One explanation for the higher transplant-related mortality in earlier bone marrow transplants appears to be delayed transplantation. The median time from diagnosis to transplant was 14 months during the first time period, but only 10 months during the later one. Other explanations might be the use of new drugs and optimization of treatment for bacterial, viral, and fungal infections. The rates of death due to interstitial pneumonitis, as well as to bacterial and fungal infections, were reduced during the later period.

Allogeneic transplantation appears to more often induce a molecular remission, which is more sustained than that following autologous transplantation. Corradini et al[16] reported that, out of 36 patients who achieved a complete remission (out of 51 patients in total), 29 were analysed for persistence of clonal cells with patient-specific clonal markers based upon the rearrangement of immunoglobulin heavy-chain genes. Fifteen of the patients underwent autologous transplantation and 14 allogeneic transplantation. Only one of the autologous patients but seven of the allogeneic ones achieved a molecular remission.

In an EBMT study, syngeneic transplantation was compared with both autologous and allogeneic transplantation.[17] Case-matching was made for the most important prognostic factors, and the 25 patients who had received a syngeneic transplant and were reported to the EBMT registry were compared with 125 autologous and 125 allogeneic case-matched transplants. Syngeneic transplantation was the most successful transplantation procedure, with an overall median survival of 72 months. It was significantly superior to allogeneic transplantation and tended to be superior to autologous transplantation. The relapse rate was similar to that with allogeneic transplantation and lower than that with autologous transplantation, and there was no significant difference in transplant-related mortality between autologous and syngeneic transplantation. In three syngeneic patients, there were signs of graft-versus-host disease (GvHD), which is still unexplained but has been described previously in syngeneic transplantation for other disorders. Syngeneic transplantation seems to be an indication for all patients below 60–65 years of age who are fortunate enough to have an identical twin.

Non-myeloablative transplantation

The concept of non-myeloablative conditioning followed by allogeneic transplantation is based on observations that engraftment can occur without myeloablation. Also, the graft will not immediately induce full chimerism, but successively with time will induce first mixed chimerism and later full chimerism. In a recent study, six myeloma patients received 200 cGy total-body irradiation as conditioning for the transplant and immunosuppression with mycophenilate mofetil plus cyclosporin.[18] The patients had previously received an autologous transplant. PBSC were obtained from HLA-matched sibling donors. Five patients are alive after a follow-up of 75–238 days. Only three patients had moderate GvHD (grade II), while two patients had no GvHD. Hospitalization was short. Thus, non-myeloablative conditioning followed by allogeneic transplantation appears to be a promising treatment approach.

NEW TREATMENTS – THALIDOMIDE

Thalidomide is an immunomodulatory drug that can inhibit angiogenesis and induce apoptosis of established neovasculature in experimental models. In multiple myeloma, there is increased vascularization, which correlates positively with a high plasma cell labeling index. In 1965, Olson et al[19] reported a positive effect on disease progression in one patient with multiple myeloma. However, this did not result in any further attempts to use thalidomide for the treatment of multiple myeloma until recently. Singhal et al[20] treated 84 previously treated patients with refractory myeloma with thalidomide. The starting dose was 200 mg per day and the dose was increased by 200 mg every two weeks up to 800 mg per day. In eight patients, serum and urine levels of paraprotein were reduced by at least 90%, in six patients, they were reduced by 75%, in seven by 50%, and in six by 25%; i.e. there was a response rate of 32%. Plasma cells were reduced in bone marrow, and hemoglobin levels increased. Thus, thalidomide has a clear effect on patients with multiple myeloma. The drug is now in trial in combinations with other drugs for conditioning of patients before autologous transplantation as well as for treatment of refractory patients. Upfront thalidomide studies will probably soon be started.

CONCLUSIONS AND OUTLOOK FOR THE FUTURE

In 1999, multiple myeloma research advanced considerably. Knowledge has increased concerning the interaction between various cytokines and signaling proteins, and in particular their interactions leading to induction or suppression of IL-6. The importance of KSHV/HHV8 is not yet settled. Further studies are needed in order to confirm that dendritic cells are infected by KSHV in myeloma, and if so, whether KSHV infection of dendritic cells has an impact on IL-6 production and thus may be of importance in the etiology and pathogenesis of the disease.

Autologous transplantation is a cornerstone in the treatment of patients below 65 years of age. Selection of CD34$^+$ cells is feasible, but there is no proof that such selection will improve survival or relapse-free survival. Tandem transplants may marginally improve results. However, second transplants may as well be performed later in the course of the disease as in close tandem with the first transplantation.

Allogeneic transplantation has improved dramatically during the last five years. Molecular remissions are more often obtained with allogeneic transplantation than with autologous transplantation, and there may be cures using allogeneic transplantation. Peripheral blood stem cell transplantation results appear to be similar to those with bone marrow. Syngeneic transplantation, when possible, appears to be the best choice. Recent non-myeloablative transplants following autologous transplantation are encouraging, and, combined with donor lymphocyte transfusion, may prove to be important in the future.

Antiangiogenic treatment is a new approach in multiple myeloma, and may well prove to be a breakthrough.

REFERENCES

1. Tarte K, Chang Y, Klein B, Kaposi's sarcoma-associated herpesvirus and multiple myeloma: lack of criteria for causality. *Blood* 1999; **93**: 3159–63.

2. Sitas F, Carrara H, Beral V et al, Antibodies against human herpesvirus 8 in black South African patients with cancer. *N Engl J Med* 1999; **340**: 1863–71.

3. Rettig MB, Ma HJ, Vescio RA et al, Kaposi's sarcoma associated herpes virus infection of bone marrow dendritic cells from multiple myeloma patients. *Science* 1997; **276**: 1851–4.

4. Chauhan D, Bharti A, Raje N et al, Detection of Kaposi's sarcoma herpesvirus DNA sequences in multiple myeloma bone marrow stromal cells. *Blood* 1999; **93**: 1482–6.

5. Berenson JR, Vescio RA, HHV-8 is present in multiple myeloma patients. *Blood* 1999; **93**: 3157–9 [discussion 3164-6].

6. Bergsagel PL, Chesi M, Kuel WM, Myeloma – a multistep transformation process. In: *Proceedings of VII International Multiple Myeloma Workshop, Stockholm* 1999: I 11.

7. Barlogie N, Jagannath S, Desikan KR et al, Total therapy with tandem transplants for newly diagnosed multiple myeloma. *Blood* 1999; **93**: 55–65.

8. Avet-Loiseau H, Li JY, Morineau N et al, Monosomy 13 is associated with the transition of monoclonal gammopathy of undetermined significance to multiple myeloma. Intergroupe Francophone du Myélome. *Blood* 1999; **94**: 2583–9.

9. Thunberg U, Banghagen M, Bengtsson M et al, Linear reduction of clonal cells in stem cell enriched grafts in transplanted multiple myeloma. *Br J Haematol* 1999; **104**: 546–52.

10. Gandhi M, Jestice H, Scott M et al, A comparison of CD34+ cell selected and unselected autologous peripheral blood stem cell transplantation for multiple myeloma: a case controlled analysis. *Bone Marrow Transplant* 1999; **24**: 369–75.

11. Vescio R, Schiller G, Stewart AK et al, Multicenter phase III trial to evaluate CD34(+) selected versus unselected autologous peripheral blood progenitor cell transplantation in multiple myeloma. *Blood* 1999; **93**: 1858–68.

12. Facon T, Harousseau JL, Maloisel F et al, Stem cell factor in combination with filgrastim after chemotherapy improves peripheral blood progenitor cell yield and reduced apheresis requirements in multiple myeloma patients: a randomized, controlled trial. *Blood* 1999; **94**: 1218–25.

13. Morris T, Svensson H, Björkstrand B, Gahrton G, Double autologous cell transplantation: effect of timing in patients with multiple myeloma. An EBMT Registry study. In: *Proceedings of VII International Multiple Myeloma Workshop, Stockholm*, 1999: P126.

14. Attal M, Harousseau JL, Facon T et al, Single versus double transplant in myeloma: a randomized trial of the 'Inter Groupe Français du Myélome' (IFM). *Blood* 1999; **94**: 714a.

15. Gahrton G, Allogeneic bone marrow transplantation in multiple myeloma. *Pathol Biol (Paris)* 1999; **47**: 188–91.

16. Corrandini P, Voena C, Tarella C et al, Molecular and clinical remissions in multiple myeloma: role of autologous and allogeneic transplantation of hematopoietic cells. *J Clin Oncol* 1999; **17**: 208–15.

17. Gahrton G, Svensson H, Björkstrand B et al, Syngeneic transplantation in multiple myeloma – a case-matched comparison with autologous and allogeneic transplantation. *Bone Marrow Transplant* 1999; **24**: 741–5.

18. Molina A, McSweeney P, Maloney DG et al, Non myeloablative peripheral blood stem cell (PBSC) allografts follow-

ing cytoreductive autotransplants for treatment of multiple myeloma (MM). *Blood* 1999; **94**: 347a.

19. Olson KB, Hall TC, Horton J et al, Thalidomide (N-phthaloylglutamimide) in the treatment of advanced cancer. *Clin Pharmacol Ther* 1965; **6**: 292–7.

20. Singhal S, Mehta J, Desikan R et al, Antitumor activity of thalidomide in refractory multiple myeloma. *N Engl J Med* 1999; **341**: 1565–71.

12

Positron emission tomography in the management of lymphomas

Paul N Mainwaring, Adrian R Timothy

INTRODUCTION

With changes in diagnostic classification systems, the introduction of new imaging techniques, and the use of more systemic therapy over the past decade, there has been a steady move away from surgical staging towards the use of other prognostic indicators for determining the optimum management of patients with lymphoma.[1,2] Nonetheless, clinical stage remains an important prognostic indicator, and will still influence the constitution and intensity of initial treatment. While computed tomography (CT) scanning is currently the most widely used imaging technique in staging and remission assessment, the introduction of functional imaging now offers the opportunity to detect sites of active disease on the basis of metabolic rather than anatomical change. Gallium-67 (^{67}Ga) scintigraphy has been available for many years for clinical use, and there is now an extensive literature on this technique in both pre-treatment staging and post-treatment assessment of patients with lymphoma. Despite the wealth of experience, however, the use of gallium scanning in routine management varies greatly from centre to centre, reflecting some of the problems with this technique. More recently, positron emission tomography (PET) using [^{18}F]2-fluoro-2-deoxy-D-glucose (^{18}FDG) has been introduced into clinical practice. There is a growing body of data suggesting not only that this is an extremely sensitive method for detecting lymphoma but also that it has advantages over both CT and gallium. This chapter will focus on improvements in our understanding of the role of PET in managing patients with lymphoma, including recently published data. It will examine the role of PET in the staging of non-Hodgkin's lymphoma (NHL) and Hodgkin's disease, and in the assessment of response to treatment, including the evaluation of residual masses, and it will compare the sensitivity and specificity of ^{18}FDG PET with gallium-67 scanning.

TECHNIQUES

The basis of PET scanning lies on the fact that most malignant tumours, including lymphomas, demonstrate increased rates of aerobic glycolysis compared with normal tissues. [18]FDG enters the cancer cell via cell membrane glucose transport proteins (e.g. GLUT1), and is phosphorylated to [18]FDG-6-phosphate by hexokinase. Although [18]FDG-6-phosphate can be dephosphorylated by glucose-6-phosphatase, this occurs slowly – particularly in cancer cells, which often lack this enzyme – and as [18]FDG-6-phosphate does not easily cross cell membranes, it becomes concentrated within the cancer cells.[3] In the setting of an elevated blood glucose level, [18]FDG uptake is reduced owing to direct competition with glucose, with loss of sensitivity of PET scanning.[4] In a normal [18]FDG PET scan, high uptake is seen in the brain and myocardium owing to their inherent high glucose metabolism, but, unlike glucose, there is excretion via the urinary tract (Figure 12.1). [18]FDG has no known side-effects and the radiation dose is similar to other nuclear medicine procedures or CT.

[18]FDG has a half-life of approximately 2 hours, and decays by emission of a positron, which at the end of its range of less than 1 mm, undergoes annihilation with an electron. This annihilation generates two 511 keV γ-rays emitted at 180° to each other, which are detected almost simultaneously (or 'in coincidence') by the circular array of the PET scanner scintillation detectors. If both γ-rays are detected within a short time of one another, it is assumed that they originated from the same annihilation event. The original disintegration occurs along a line joining the two detection positions; upon reconstruction, this will give a very accurate picture of the site, and, owing to the ability to accurately correct for photon attenuation within the body, PET offers a good degree of accuracy within the area of interest.

The half-life of [18]FDG permits acquisition of whole-body images over approximately 60 minutes. The axial field of view of most PET scanners is limited to approximately 15 cm, and so, in order to scan larger areas, the patient is moved through the gantry on a couch, creating a trade-off between longer scanning times for increased accuracy against patients' ability to remain comfortable and lie still.

Owing to the expense of a full-dedicated whole-body PET scanner and the introduction of coincidence electronics in conventional gamma cameras, the possibility of extending double-headed cameras for PET use has been explored. Unfortunately, the decreased count-rate capability of hybrid PET/SPECT (single-photon emission CT) cameras may reduce the ability to detect small lesions. In compensation for this, hybrid PET/SPECT equipment uses a much larger field of view, and the imaging may need to be conducted over a much longer time.[4] Naumann and colleagues[5] undertook a comparison of both techniques in 16 patients with Hodgkin's disease and 4 with NHL at time of initial staging and recurrence, and also for residual disease assessment. The reduced sensitivity of the dual-headed camera was reflected in a lower rate of detection

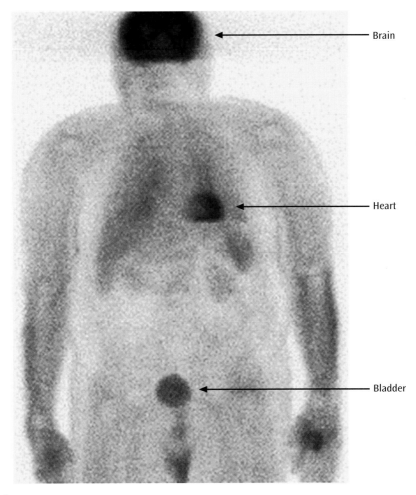

Figure 12.1
Normal whole-body ¹⁸FDG PET scan, showing uptake in brain, heart, kidneys and bladder.

of both nodal and extranodal disease, as well as resulting in inaccurate staging in 3 of 13 patients.

STAGING

Traditionally, lymphoma staging has used the Ann Arbor classification system, which is based on clinical and radiological features.[6,7] Over the last decade, improvements in non-invasive imaging techniques have resulted in the suggestion that the results from CT scanning, magnetic resonance imaging (MRI) scanning, and gallium-67 imaging be included as additional criteria for staging.[8] Posterior iliac crest bone marrow biopsy remains an important part of the diagnostic work-up, with bilateral sampling providing better sensitivity than a single aspirate and trephine sample.[9] Clinical and pathological staging continue to have prognostic significance, and influence treatment strategies in the majority of patients despite the increased use of systemic therapy.

CT scanning uses morphological changes and size criteria as a possible indicator of disease activity.[10] As such, CT scanning is inherently limited in its ability (1) to detect active disease in normal sized lymph nodes, (2) to detect active disease in lymph nodes that may have increased in size in response to other causes, (3) to assess disease activity in both liver and spleen, and (4) to differentiate between post-treatment fibrosis and active disease in residual masses.

Clinical research over the last several years has consistently shown that PET scanning is more sensitive than CT scanning in determining sites of active disease in heterogeneous populations of lymphoma patients.[11–14] PET scanning was compared with CT and MRI as well as with gallium-67 scanning and lymphangiography by Hoh et al.[12] In this study, whole-body PET was accurate in staging 17 of 18 patients, identifying additional disease in 5 of 18 patients, including extranodal sites. However, [18]FDG PET failed to demonstrate histologically proven sites of disease in 2 patients. Moog and colleagues[15,16] have extended their initial investigations into the role of PET in the assessment of extranodal lymphoma, and have reported PET to be sensitive, with fewer false positives than CT, in identifying sites of extranodal disease, including bone marrow, spleen, liver, and lung.

If the assumption that whole-body [18]FDG PET has increased sensitivity in detecting lymphoma is correct, the question is then raised as to how this impacts on clinical management. Stage migration is a common problem with the introduction of new technologies. Jerusalem and colleagues[17] have recently reported their investigation of [18]FDG PET in staging 60 patients with varying histological subtypes, some of whom were investigated at first presentation and others at time of relapse. Although more lymph node sites were identified by [18]FDG PET in 15 patients, stage changed in only 2 patients, and this change did not influence subsequent treatment. In the comparison of extranodal disease, there was reported discordance between [18]FDG PET and clinical examination/CT scanning in 5 of 15 patients; however, in only 1 patient was this discrepancy confirmed histologically.

From our own unpublished data on 44 patients with Hodgkin's disease, 159 sites of disease involvement were demonstrated with [18]FDG PET, compared with 84 by CT scanning. In this patient population, 41% of patients were upstaged, many because of extranodal disease not visualized by CT. Three patients were downstaged by PET, and in 11/44 (25%) patients, treatment would have been modified as a consequence of the PET findings.[18]

In an attempt to further improve the diagnostic accuracy of [18]FDG PET in lymphoma, Kotzerke and colleagues[19] have investigated the role of attenuation correction in the detection of nodal and extranodal sites of disease. Two independent observers using a visual intensity scale assessed [18]FDG PET-positive nodal regions in 51 patients. All 37 extranodal sites were detected with equal sensitivity by both attenuation-corrected or uncorrected images. In 24 nodal sites, there was uncertainty about the cause of increased [18]FDG uptake, and in only 5 of 24 sites was attenuation correction helpful in differentiating malignant from 'equivocal' uptake as perceived by the investigators. While this was only a small study, there is little evidence from these data to suggest that further investigation of the role of attenuation correction is likely to yield much benefit in whole-body [18]FDG PET assessment for lymphoma staging. Nor does the study suggest that PET is sufficiently accurate at the present time to eliminate the need for concomitant CT or MRI scanning. As not all sites of extranodal disease were confirmed histologically, the changes in [18]FDG uptake following treatment may have been used as an additional indicator of the accuracy of PET in identifying disease.

In a study from the University of Ulm comparing conventional technetium bone scanning and [18]FDG PET, 12 of 56 patients were identified as having skeletal involvement by lymphoma, confirmed by CT, MRI, plain radiography, or biopsy.[20] Both PET and bone scanning identified areas of involvement, confirmed by biopsy, despite negative staging bone marrow examinations. PET scanning identified more sites of active disease than technetium in concordant patients, as well as identifying sites of bony disease in 5 patients with negative technetium scans. In a further 5 patients where the bone scan was positive and [18]FDG PET-negative, further investigation showed that none of these abnormalities was due to lymphoma. This study highlights the potential biological differences between focal and diffuse lymphomatous involvement, with possible implications for pre-treatment staging and prognosis. This study also emphasizes the need for histological confirmation in areas of doubt in order to truly define the positive and negative predictive value of whole-body [18]FDG PET scanning.

Moog et al[21] have also reported a comparison of [18]FDG PET with bone marrow aspirate and trephine in staging 78 untreated patients with either NHL ($n = 39$) or Hodgkin's disease ($n = 39$). Biopsy revealed 4 cases of bone marrow involvement not detectable by [18]FDG PET scanning (5.1%), with concordant results in 64 patients (82%). [18]FDG PET showed uptake suggesting bone marrow involvement in 10 patients with negative bone marrow examinations (12.8%). In 8 out of the 10 cases, the [18]FDG PET findings were confirmed by other modalities. The authors concluded that the [18]FDG PET scans provided additional information leading to an upgrade of the tumour stage in 10.3% (8 of 78) of patients. Similarly, Carr et al[22] have previously published results suggesting that visual abnormalities on [18]FDG PET correlate accurately with bone marrow staging (78%), offering a potential substitute for bone marrow aspirate and trephine. In 8 (16%) of the remaining patients, [18]FDG PET-positive and bone marrow-negative disease was reported, and, despite further attempts to resolve the causes for the discrepancy between the two techniques, this could not be resolved in 5 (10%).

Table 12.1 Comparison of ¹⁸FDG PET and gallium-67 scanning

¹⁸FDG PET	⁶⁷Gallium
High-resolution – 3D image reconstruction	Lower resolution – need for SPECT
Low gastrointestinal uptake	High gastrointestinal uptake
Short scanning time (approx. 2 hours)	Delayed images required (several days)
Half-life 110 minutes	Half-life 72 hours
Average whole-body exposure approx. 9 mSv	Average whole body exposure approx. 18 mSv (whole-body CT scan approx. 27 mSv)

By contrast, Jerusalem and colleagues[17] could support the case for ¹⁸PET FDG as a substitute for bone marrow aspirate and trephine according to the results of their study. Bone marrow infiltration was suggested in 18 of 60 patients on ¹⁸FDG PET (16 focal, 2 diffuse). Marrow infiltration was confirmed in 13 of 18, biopsy was negative in 4, and in 1 patient it was not performed. Therefore, at least 4 of 18 (22%) patients would have been incorrectly upstaged. In 8 other patients (13%) in whom ¹⁸FDG PET did not suggest bone marrow infiltration, bone marrow biopsy confirmed active disease, suggesting that these patients were incorrectly downstaged.

Gallium-67 scanning is regularly used by many institutions for staging lymphoma; however, its role remains controversial. Comparison of the essential features of gallium-67 and ¹⁸FDG PET scanning are summarized in Table 12.1 In essence, ¹⁸FDG PET has several advantages when compared with gallium-67. Furthermore, the problems of gut contamination with gallium mean that it is an unreliable investigation for detecting sub-diaphragmetic disease. In contrast with gallium-67, ¹⁸FDG PET appears to be more sensitive than CT both above and below the diaphragm.[12,18,23] In a study of 33 patients, direct comparison was made with ¹⁸FDG PET using a dual-headed coincident camera with attentuation correction and gallium-67 scintigraphy.[24] FDG PET was positive in all 33 patients, compared with only 24 positive scans with gallium-67. CT and clinical correlation of these sites confirmed the accuracy of the additional PET findings in all 9 patients. The authors conclude that in pre-treatment staging of lymphoma, ¹⁸FDG PET was significantly more sensitive and accurate than gallium-67 scanning. Given the uncertainty expressed about the specificity of PET or gallium-67 every effort should be made to biopsy suspicious sites where appropriate.

Summary

On the present evidence, [18]FDG PET is consistently more accurate in the detection of nodal and extranodal sites of lymphoma compared with CT, MRI, or gallium-67. The impact on staging and subsequent treatment remains unresolved at this time, however, and much further work is required in more homogeneous patient populations. For the present, conventional staging techniques remain the gold standard.

REMISSION AND RESPONSE ASSESSMENT

As well as demonstrating a role in staging patients with lymphoma, changes in the qualitative and quantitative parameters of whole-body [18]FDG PET may have the ability to predict response to treatment. Recently, the EORTC PET group has made recommendations on the measurement of [18]FDG uptake for tumour response, which have yet to be assessed prospectively in managing patients with lymphoma.[25] In a small study from Munich, [18]FDG PET was used to assess 11 patients with high-grade NHL for their response to combination chemotherapy at 7 and 42 days after treatment.[26] They observed that the maximal reduction in the quantitative values occurred between these two time points and that response could be correlated with the reduction in [18]FDG PET uptake measured at day 42. Our own data suggest that an interim PET scan after two cycles of chemotherapy is an accurate predictor of failure-free survival, and is more sensitive than [18]FDG PET scanning performed at completion of treatment.[27] This is consistent with the data from the study by Janicek and colleagues[28] and the more recent data from Front and colleagues,[29] who have shown that a gallium-67 scan repeated after one cycle of chemotherapy is an excellent prognostic indicator for failure-free survival in those patients whose gallium-67 scan becomes negative compared to those patients where there is persistent gallium-67 activity ($p = 0.0005$).

RESIDUAL MASS

At the completion of conventional treatment, residual abnormalities on CT or plain X-ray present a therapeutic dilemma. While less than one-quarter of patients with a residual mass following treatment will relapse,[30] accurate assessment of response to treatment in lymphoma is essential to differentiate those patients in whom disease has not been irradicated and who require further therapy from those in complete remission in whom further treatment is unnecessary and may only increase morbidity. There is increasing concern about late morbidity following treatment for Hodgkin's disease, particularly with the use of chemotherapy and mediastinal radiation with regard to breast carcinoma in young women and cardiac disease in young males.[31] If it is possible to accurately define complete remission following chemotherapy, mediastinal radiation might be avoided, with the benefits of reduced toxicity.

There are a limited number of reports of [18]FDG PET in the evaluation of residual masses posttreatment. De Wit et al,[32] in a study of 27 patients with Hodgkin's disease and NHL, showed that 7 out of 10 who were PET-positive following treatment relapsed, compared with none out of 17 who were PET-negative. Follow-up of this study was, however, short (60 weeks), and a further update is awaited. In their retrospective analysis of 72 patients with mixed histologies, Crimerius and colleagues[33] compared PET, CT, and lactate dehydrogenase (LDH) level for their value in assessing residual masses. PET had a sensitivity of 88%, a specificity of 83%, and an overall accuracy of 85%, with CT scanning having values of 84%, 31%, and 54%, and LDH having values of 50%, 92%, and 73%, respectively. Jerusalem and colleagues[23] have reported on the role of whole-body [18]FDG PET in discriminating persistent disease in residual masses in 54 patients with aggressive NHL or Hodgkin's disease 1–3 months after the completion of treatment. All 6 patients with a positive [18]FDG PET scan relapsed; however, 8 of 48 (17%) [18]FDG PET-negative residual masses also relapsed. PET was therefore superior in identifying risk of relapse than evidence of a residual mass on CT. Progression-free and overall survival were best for patients with negative studies (87% progression-free survival at two years), intermediate for patients with negative PET scans and a residual mass on CT (60% progression-free survival at two years), and worst when both studies were positive (no progression-free survival at two years). This is a landmark paper that raises further questions as to the sensitivity and specificity of these investigations and the most appropriate timing. The observation that some patients relapsed outside known sites of disease underlines the limitations of both techniques. Better correlation between negative PET, cross-sectional imaging, and molecular assessment of 'minimal residual disease' to improve accuracy is the next logical step in this area.

Mikhaeel and colleagues,[27] in a study of 32 patients with NHL and Hodgkin's disease and with a median follow-up of 38 months, have also demonstrated that patients with a persistent mediastinal mass on CT and a positive PET scan have a high risk (89%) of relapse compared with those whose [18]FDG PET scan becomes negative (9%) after treatment.

In a study of ^{67}Ga SPECT in patients with residual mediastinal masses on CT scanning, Zinzani and colleagues[34] reported that 100% (3 of 3) patients with a negative CT and positive gallium-67 scan relapsed, compared with only 6% (1 of 18) patients when the gallium-67 scan was negative. In 54 patients with positive restaging CT scans, 13 also had positive gallium-67 scans; 10 (77%) of these relapsed. This compares with only 5 of 41 (12%) patients with a negative gallium-67 but 'positive' CT scan. Kostakoglu and colleagues[24] have reported a comparative study of [18]FDG PET (dual-head coincidence camera with attenuation correction) and gallium-67 scanning post therapy. There was discordance in 6 of 46 (13%) patients: 3 with negative [18]FDG PET and positive gallium-67 scans and 3 vice versa. Unfortunately, no follow-up data are yet available from this study, which might improve our understanding of the reasons for discordance between these two types of functional imaging.

Summary

From the limited data available, [18]FDG PET is at least equivalent to gallium-67 in detecting disease in residual masses and as a prognostic indicator for relapse following treatment. Larger numbers and longer follow-up are required. Advances in PET technology are currently being evaluated, and may permit further improvements in diagnostic accuracy.

PITFALLS

[18]FDG PET is probably the most sensitive technique currently available for detecting Hodgkin's disease and NHL; however, PET-scan results must be viewed in the context of clinical examination, and other imaging and laboratory investigations. As with any other technique [18]FDG PET is not infallible. In Figure 12.2, a patient with biopsy-proven diffuse large B-cell NHL with extensive axillary lymphadenopathy on CT scanning, but a totally negative PET scan, is shown. Similarly, Figure 12.3 shows a [18]FDG PET scan in a patient who presented with fever, night sweats, and lymphadenopathy four months after achieving complete remission following treatment for diffuse large B-cell NHL as judged by clinical, CT, and PET criteria. This scan shows uptake in peripheral lymph node groups suggestive of recurrent NHL; however, the patient had rising varicella zoster virus titres and subsequently developed clinical signs of varicella zoster. When the titres and clinical signs resolved, the [18]FDG PET scan returned to normal. This patient remains in remission 18 months post therapy.

SUMMARY

[18]FDG PET is a very exciting tool for the assessment of disease extent and response to treatment in lymphoma. For centres fortunate to have access to [18]FDG PET scanning facilities, this is increasingly being integrated into routine management. There remain many unresolved issues, however, and further well-conducted collaborative clinical studies in homogeneous patient populations are needed to fully assess the potential benefits for the patient. These studies should also include a detailed analysis of the cost-effectiveness of [18]FDG PET.

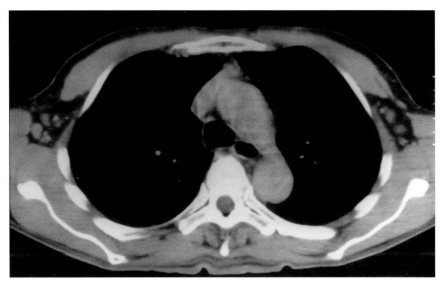

(a)

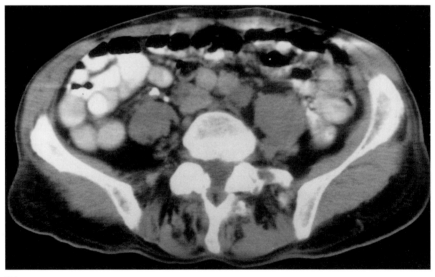

(b)

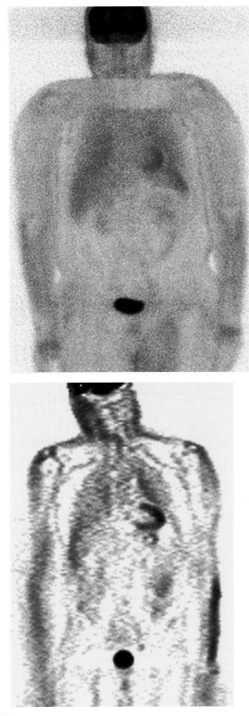

(c)

Figure 12.2

Negative [18]FDG PET scan in a patient with clinical stage III diffuse large B-cell NHL: (a) CT scan demonstrating axillary lymphadenopathy; (b) CT scan demonstrating para-aortic lymphadenopathy; (c) negative [18]FDG PET scan despite disease demonstrated in (a) and (b).

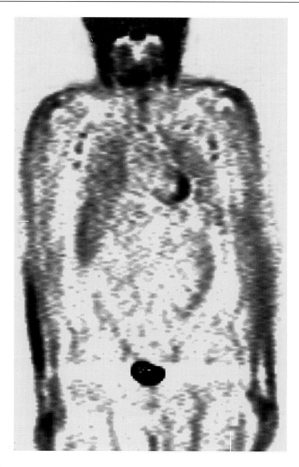

Figure 12.3

Positive [18]FDG PET uptake in axillary lymph nodes in a patient in complete remission post chemotherapy for diffuse large B-cell NHL with varicella zoster infection.

ACKNOWLEDGEMENTS

We are indebted to Dr Gray Cook for his checking of the techniques section of this manuscript and to Mrs Bernadette Cronin for help with the PET images.

REFERENCES

1 Tubiana M, Henry-Amar M, Carde P et al, Toward comprehensive management tailored to prognostic factors of patients with clinical stages I and II in Hodgkin's disease. The EORTC Lymphoma Group controlled clinical trials: 1964–1987. *Blood* 1989; **73**: 47–56.

2. The International Non-Hodgkin's Lymphoma Prognostic Factors Project, A predictive model for aggressive non-Hodgkin's lymphoma. *N Engl J Med* 1993; **329**: 987–94.

3. Maisey MN, Wahl RL, Barrington SF, Oncology: a brief overview. In: *Atlas of Clinical Positron Emission Tomography* (Maisey MN, Wahl RL, Barrington SF, eds). London: Arnold, 1999.

4. Harolds JA, 18-Fluorodeoxyglucose imaging in oncology. *J Okla State Med Assoc* 1999; **92**: 457–61.

5. Naumann R, Schirmer L, Tiepolt C et al, PET for evaluation of tumor metabolism in malignant lymphomas – optimization of the cost-benefit. *Blood* 1999; **94** (Suppl 1): A4325.

6. Rosenberg SA, Boiron M, DeVita Jr VT et al, Report of the Committee on Hodgkin's Disease Staging Procedures. *Cancer Res* 1971; **31**: 1862–3.

7. Carbone PP, Kaplan HS, Musshoff K et al, Report of the Committee on Hodgkin's Disease Staging Classification. *Cancer Res* 1971; **31**: 1860–1.

8. Lister TA, Crowther D, Sutcliffe SB et al, Report of a committee convened to discuss the evaluation and staging of patients with Hodgkin's disease: Cotswolds meeting. *J Clin Oncol* 1989; **7**: 1630–6.

9. Brunning RD, Bloomfield CD, McKenna RW et al, Bilateral trephine bone marrow biopsies in lymphoma and other neoplastic diseases. *Ann Intern Med* 1975; **82**: 365–6.

10. Cheson BD, Horning SJ, Coiffier B et al, Report of an international workshop to standardize response criteria for non-Hodgkin's lymphomas. *J Clin Oncol* 1999; **17**: 1244.

11. Timothy AR, Ahern V, Barrington S et al, FDG PET scanning in staging and remission assessment of malignant lymphoma. In: *Proceedings of International Conference on Lymphoma, Lugarno, Switzerland, 1996.*

12. Hoh CK, Glaspy J, Rosen P et al, Whole-body FDG-PET imaging for staging of Hodgkin's disease and lymphoma. *J Nucl Med* 1997; **38**: 343–8.

13. Bangerter M, Moog F, Buchmann I et al, Whole-body 2-[^{18}F]-fluoro-2-deoxy-D-glucose positron emission tomography (FDG-PET) for accurate staging of Hodgkin's disease. *Ann Oncol* 1998; **9**: 1117–22.

14. Stumpe KD, Urbinelli M, Steinert HC et al, Whole-body positron emission tomography using fluorodeoxyglucose for staging of lymphoma: effectiveness and comparison with computed tomography. *Eur J Nucl Med* 1998; **25**: 721–8.

15. Moog F, Bangerter M, Diederichs CG et al, Lymphoma: role of whole-body 2-deoxy-2-[F-18]fluoro-D-glucose (FDG) PET in nodal staging. *Radiology* 1997; **203**: 795–800.

16. Moog F, Bangerter M, Diederichs CG et al, Extranodal malignant lymphoma: detection with FDG PET versus CT. *Radiology* 1998; **206**: 475–81.

17. Jerusalem G, Warland V, Najjar F et al, Whole-body ^{18}F-FDG PET for the evaluation of patients with Hodgkin's disease and non-Hodgkin's lymphoma. *Nucl Med Commun* 1999; **20**: 13–20.

18. Partridge S, 2-Fluorine-18-fluoro-2-deoxy-D-glucose positron emission tomography in the pretreatment staging of Hodgkin's disease. *Ann Oncol* 2000; in press.

19. Kotzerke J, Guhlmann A, Moog F et al, Role of attenuation correction for fluorine-18 fluorodeoxyglucose positron emission tomography in the primary staging of malignant lymphoma. *Eur J Nucl Med* 1999; **26**: 31–8.

20. Moog F, Kotzerke J, Reske SN, FDG PET can replace bone scintigraphy in

primary staging of malignant lymphoma. *J Nucl Med* 1999; **40**: 1407–13.

21. Moog F, Bangerter M, Kotzerke J et al, 18-F-fluorodeoxyglucose–positron emission tomography as a new approach to detect lymphomatous bone marrow. *J Clin Oncol* 1998; **16**: 603–9.

22. Carr R, Barrington SF, Madan B et al, Detection of lymphoma in bone marrow by whole-body positron emission tomography. *Blood* 1998; **91**: 3340–6.

23. Jerusalem G, Beguin Y, Fassotte MF et al, Whole-body positron emission tomography using ^{18}F-fluorodeoxyglucose for posttreatment evaluation in Hodgkin's disease and non-Hodgkin's lymphoma has higher diagnostic and prognostic value than classical computed tomography scan imaging. *Blood* 1999; **94**: 429–33.

24. Kostakoglu L, Leonard JP, Coleman M et al, Comparison of fluorine-18 fluorodeoxyglucose positron emission tomography (FDG-PET) and gallium-67 scintigraphy in staging and follow-up of patients with lymphoma. *Blood* 1999; **94** (Suppl 1): A365.

25. Young H, Baum R, Cremerius U et al, Measurement of clinical and subclinical tumour response using [^{18}F]-fluorodeoxyglucose and positron emission tomography: review and 1999 EORTC recommendations. European Organization for Research and Treatment of Cancer (EORTC) PET Study Group. *Eur J Cancer* 1999; **35**: 1773–82.

26. Romer W, Hanauske AR, Ziegler S et al, Positron emission tomography in non-Hodgkin's lymphoma: assessment of chemotherapy with flurodeoxyglucose. *Blood* 1998; **91**: 4464–71.

27. Mikhaeel NG, Timothy AR, Hain SF, O'Doherty MJ, 18-FDG-PET for the assessment of residual masses on CT following treatment of lymphomas. *Ann Oncol* 2000; **11** (Suppl 1): S147–50.

28. Janicek M, Kaplan W, Neuberg D et al, Early restaging gallium scans predict outcome in poor-prognosis patients with aggressive non-Hodgkin's lymphoma treated with high-dose CHOP chemotherapy. *J Clin Oncol* 1997; **15**: 1631–7.

29. Front D, Bar-Shalom R, Mor M et al, Prediction of outcome of patients with Hodgkin's disease (HD) by GA-67 scintigraphy after one cycle of chemotherapy. *J Nucl Med* 1998; **39** (Suppl 5): 10P.

30. Canellos GP, Residual mass in lymphoma may not be residual disease. *J Clin Oncol* 1988; **6**: 931–3.

31. Donaldson SS, Hancock SL, Hoppe RT, The Janeway Lecture. Hodgkin's disease – finding the balance between cure and late effects. *Cancer J Sci Am* 1999; **5**: 325–33.

32. De Wit M, Bumann D, Beyer W et al, Whole-body positron emission tomography (PET) for diagnosis of residual mass in patients with lymphoma. *Ann Oncol* 1997; **8** (Suppl 1): 57–60.

33. Cremerius U, Fabry U, Kroll U et al, Clinical value of FDG-PET for therapy monitoring of malignant lymphoma – results of a retrospective study in 72 patients. *Nuklearmedizin* 1999; **38**: 24–30.

34. Zinzani PL, Magagnoli M, Franchi R et al, Diagnostic role of gallium scanning in the management of lymphoma with mediastinal involvement. *Haematologica* 1999; **84**: 604–7.

13
Monoclonal antibodies have finally arrived

Jennifer B Lucas, Sandra J Horning

INTRODUCTION

One century ago, Paul Erlich postulated that antibodies could prove to be the 'magic bullets' of cancer therapy.[1] The arrival of monoclonal antibodies (MoAbs) for the treatment of cancer has long been anticipated, and significant advances in the development and clinical application of MoAbs have occurred. The feasibility of passive immunotherapy became practical when Kohler and Milstein[2] reported the fusion of a mouse myeloma cell with a mouse splenocyte from an immunized donor, resulting in a hybridoma capable of producing specific MoAbs. The advantages of MoAbs over conventional therapy are numerous, and include the delivery of a targeted therapy, recruitment of the host immune system, avoidance of chemotherapy- or radiation-associated toxicities, and potential enhancement of standardized therapy with combination or adjuvant approaches. Several MoAbs are now available or undergoing clinical trials for the lymphoid malignancies; however, clinicians are faced with the challenge of how to best incorporate them into the treatment regimens of these heterogeneous neoplasms.

LYMPHOID TARGET ANTIGENS

The first attempts to treat lymphoid malignancies with monoclonal antibodies began 20 years ago.[3–5] Miller and colleagues[3] reported a successful therapeutic response in a patient with relapsed follicular lymphoma using a murine monoclonal anti-idiotype antibody. Similarly, murine antibodies were used to treat T-cell malignancies, but the responses were not as durable or dramatic.[6,7]

A number of tumor surface antigens have been targeted by MoAbs for the treatment of lymphoid malignancies. While patient-specific anti-idiotype MoAbs have shown activity in follicular lymphoma in several studies, logistical difficulties and labor-intensive preparation of specific anti-idiotypes made their availability for widespread use impractical.[3,8,9] Further, the evolution of significant idiotype mutations and the circulation of free antigen often reduced the anti-tumor effect of anti-idiotype antibodies.[10] Consequently, pan-B-cell anti-gens, such as CD19, CD20, and CD22, were appreciated as more attractive tar-gets. Critical to the development of an effective antibody has been the suitable selection of an antigen that is relatively tumor-specific, present on all tumor cells with significant levels of expression, and not shed or internalized upon antibody binding. The CD20 antigen, a 35 kDa phosphoprotein, is restricted to the B-cell lineage and is expressed by mature B cells and most malignant B cell lymphomas.[11] While the exact functions of CD20 are unknown, it may play an integral role in the activation of cell cycle progression in B lymphocytes, possibly via calcium regulation.[12,13] Attractive attributes of the CD20 antigen include its tetraspan binding in the cell membrane and the lack of internaliza-tion or downregulation upon antibody binding.[14]

ANTIBODY CHARACTERISTICS

The initial trials tested murine antibodies, which proved to be immunogenic and to have a short-half life. To address these shortcomings and to elicit a more robust host immune response, chimeric and humanized antibodies were developed. Chimeric MoAbs are produced by substituting the Fc region of the murine MoAb with a human Fc portion, whereas humanized MoAbs are gener-ated by grafting the complementarity-determining region from the murine MoAb into a human antibody framework. In addition to unconjugated MoAbs, advancements in conjugation chemistry have led to the development of radio-labeled monoclonal antibodies and immunotoxins for human use.

UNCONJUGATED MONOCLONAL ANTIBODIES

Mechanism of action

In vitro data show that blockade of the receptor initiates antibody-dependent cellular cytotoxicity (ADCC) and complement-mediated lysis.[15] These cyto-toxic mechanisms depend on adequate levels of complement proteins and effector cells (granulocytes, eosinophils, and tissue macrophages), in addition to sufficient antigen-binding sites. Further clearance of circulating lymphoma cells coated with antibody is achieved by the reticuloendothelial system. There is also evidence to suggest that some MoAbs directly inhibit cellular prolifera-tion and induce apoptosis.[12,16] Understanding the mechanism(s) of action is critical to the use of MoAbs in lymphoma either as single-agents or in combi-nation with conventional therapy. Whereas the additional apoptotic signal from MoAbs argues in favor of combination strategies, immune-mediated killing requires adequate effector cells, which may be insufficient after chemotherapy. Investigations to understand mechanisms of resistance and cross-resistance to other therapies are ongoing.

Rituximab single-agent clinical trials

Rituximab, a chimeric IgG1κ monoclonal antibody that recognizes the CD20 antigen,[17] is the most widely recognized and used MoAb in the B-cell lymphoid malignancies (Table 13.1). A series of phase I/II trials determined the dosing schedule of 375 mg/m^2 weekly times four in patients with relapsed indolent non-Hodgkin's lymphoma (NHL).[11,17,18] In the multiple-dose study, three complete responses and 14 partial responses were noted in 34 evaluable patients, with a median response duration of 8.6 months. Events were primarily infusion-related toxicities (fever, headache, chills, and asthenias), with rapid and selective depletion of circulating B cells. In the phase III pivotal trial, 166 patients with relapsed indolent lymphoma were treated at a dose of 375 mg/m^2 weekly for four weeks.[19] An overall response rate of 48% was seen (6% complete and 42% partial), and in those patients who responded, the median time to progression was 13 months. Based on efficacy and safety data, the FDA approved rituximab for the treatment of relapsed or refractory indolent NHL in November 1997.

Subsequent single-agent strategies included treating patients who have previously responded to rituximab or extending the duration of treatment. In a phase II trial, 57 patients who had previously responded to rituximab were retreated.[20] At enrollment, all patients were human anti-chimeric antibody (HACA)-negative and all tumors continued to express the CD20 antigen. Although the estimated median time to progression in responders was 16.7 months, which was longer than the 12.4-month median time to progression following the initial course of rituximab, the 40% response rate suggested the acquisition of resistance. These data indicate that the benefit of repeated treatments after each relapse would be limited. Extended treatment with rituximab over eight consecutive weeks, tested in 37 patients with relapsed low-grade NHL,[21] yielded an overall response rate of 57% and an estimated time to progression of 16 months. This marginal improvement over the four-week dosing schedule in a small subset of patients treated does not justify extending treatment to eight weeks.

Because the pivotal trial excluded patients with masses larger than 10 cm, Davis et al[22] conducted a study to determine the safety and efficacy of rituximab in 37 relapsed low-grade NHL patients with bulky (mass >10 cm) disease. No patients required discontinuation of treatment due to side-effects, and the overall response rate in 28 assessable patients was 43%, with a median time to progression of 8.1 months. A lower response rate among patients with large tumors was predicted by animal studies, and presumably results from limitations in diffusion of antibody.

Owing to the toxicity of treatment and the lack of demonstrated survival benefit, asymptomatic follicular lymphoma patients are often observed without therapy. Solal-Celigny and colleagues[23] explored the role of rituximab as initial therapy in 50 untreated follicular lymphoma patients of low tumor burden, and reported an overall response rate of 69% (31% complete and 10%

Table 13.1 Rituximab treatment of B-cell malignancies

Clinical trial	Patient population[a]	ORR[b] (%)	Comments	Ref
Pivotal	166 patients with recurrent low-grade lymphoma, predominantly FSC	48 (17)	Led to FDA approval in November 1997 for use in recurrent low-grade B-cell lymphomas	19
Repeated treatment	57 patients with recurrent low-grade NHL who previously responded	40	Lower response rate suggests acquisition of resistance	20
Extended treatment	37 patients with recurrent low-grade lymphoma, treated for 8 weeks	57 (14)	Well tolerated; slightly higher overall response rate in small subset of patients does not justify extended duration	21
Bulky disease	37 relapsed low-grade NHL patients with masses >10 cm	43 (4)	Lower response rate suggests that other therapies should be considered when a brisk clinical response is desired	22
Other B-cell histologic subtypes	131 patients with MCL, IMC, and SLL	30 (<10)	Other B-cell histologies may not be as responsive to rituximab as follicular lymphoma	26
Aggressive lymphomas	54 patients with aggressive lymphoma, DLCL or MCL	32 (9)	Although well tolerated, the modest response rate argues for combination trials	27
Upfront treatment	50 asymptomatic, 'low-tumor-burden' patients	69 (31)	Disappointing complete response rate in favorable patients	23
CHOP[c] + rituximab	35 evaluable patients with intermediate- or high-grade lymphoma	100 (63)	Well-tolerated regimen with impressive overall response rate; randomized trial needed to confirm results	28
CHOP + rituximab	40 patients with recurrent low-grade NHL received 6 infusions of rituximab +6 cycles of CHOP	95 (55)	May be administered with CHOP safely; impressive overall response rate must be tempered by the small number of patients and limited follow-up to assess overall survival	29

[a]FSC, follicular small cleaved cell; MCL, mantle cell lymphoma; IMC, immunocytoma; SLL, small lymphocytic lymphoma; DLCL, diffuse large cell lymphoma.
[b]Overall response rate (complete response rate in parentheses).
[c]Cyclophosphamide, doxorubicin, vincristine, and prednisone.

complete unconfirmed using the new criteria). In this favorable patient population, the majority of patients responded; however, the responses were generally incomplete. In an ongoing trial, untreated patients are treated with rituximab on a more continuous basis. Owing to the failure of multi-agent chemotherapy to clearly improve survival in asymptomatic untreated patients, these trials should be followed with interest.

Thus far, rituximab has been most extensively tested in patients with follicular histologies, but experience in other histologic subtypes is accumulating. In the rituximab pivotal trial, it was observed that patients with a follicular histology had a superior overall response rate (69%) compared with patients with small lymphocytic lymphoma (SLL) (14%).[19] It has been postulated that the inferior response is due to the lower level of CD20 antigen expression on the cell surface and the lower serum antibody concentrations observed in these patients.[19,24,25]

Foran et al[26] treated 131 patients with mantle-cell lymphoma (MCL), immunocytoma (IMC), and SLL with standard doses of rituximab. Among the 120 assessable patients, the overall response rate was 30%. The response rates for each histology were 38% for MCL, 28% for IMC, and 14% for SLL. Among the 53 patients with IMC and SLL, none achieved a complete response. Thus, clinicians should recognize the histologic variation in response when considering treatment with rituximab.

In an intent-to-treat analysis, single-agent rituximab was used to treat 54 patients with aggressive lymphoma, the majority of whom had either diffuse large cell lymphoma (56%) or mantle cell lymphoma (24%).[27] While 17% of patients had previously untreated disease, the overall response rate was 32% in 52 evaluable patients, well below those (60–70%) obtained in commonly used salvage chemotherapy regimens.[28–30] Given the modest activity and favorable toxicity profile of rituximab in recurrent aggressive lymphomas, combination trials should be performed.

Combination clinical trials

The appreciation that most, if not all, patients with indolent lymphoma and a significant number of patients with aggressive NHL are not cured with conventional chemotherapy and/or radiotherapy has led to an explosion of clinical trials to further clarify the role of rituximab in the treatment of B-cell malignancies. The combination of its significant single-agent activity, favorable toxicity profile, and the desire to elucidate possible additive or synergistic mechanisms provides the rationale for combining rituximab with conventional therapy in a concurrent or adjuvant fashion. A small combination trial employing CHOP (cyclophosphamide, doxorubicin, vincristine, and prednisone) and rituximab concurrently for initial treatment of patients with aggressive NHL demonstrated safety.[31] Evaluation of the efficacy of combination therapy requires a comparative trial such as the Intergroup E4494 trial currently in progress. Czuczman et al[32] treated 40 patients with low-grade NHL with six infusions of rituximab in combination with six cycles of CHOP. Thirty-five patients completed the full schedule of treatment, with a response rate of 95%. Twenty-two patients (55%) experienced a complete response and 16 patients (40%) a partial response. The median time to progression had not been reached, but 70% of patients remained in remission at four years.[33] Although these results are encouraging, this study is single-armed and has small numbers of patients, with heterogeneous histologies. Further, patients with tumors larger than 10 cm were excluded, possibly selecting for more favorable outcomes. In conclusion, CHOP plus rituximab is a feasible treatment combination with acceptable toxicity, but its treatment efficacy in either indolent or aggressive B-cell lymphoma requires further clinical investigation through prospective randomized studies. Although not formally studied, we do not recommend treatment with rituximab to 'touch-up' incomplete chemotherapy responses because of the theoretical concern of induction of resistance. The combination of rituximab with purine analogs will require close observation because of the immunosuppressive effects on both the B-cell and T-cell arms of the immune system.

Rituximab adverse events

The phase III pivotal trial demonstrated that human anti-mouse antibodies (HAMA) or human anti-chimeric antibodies (HACA) occurred in less than 1% of patients, B-cell reconstitution occurred between 6–9 months, and there were no clinically apparent associated infections. The side-effects of rituximab are generally infusion-related and self-limited. During the first infusion, patients may experience fever, headache, or rigors. These symptoms subside with temporary cessation of the infusion and administration of ancillary medicines. With each subsequent treatment, there is a reduction in the infusion-related side-effects. Since the FDA approval of rituximab, additional treatment experience has amassed, and severe infusional reactions have been reported.[34] Such reactions were more common in patients with high numbers of circulating tumor cells in the peripheral blood, and manifest as severe rigors, fever, bronchospasm, hypoxemia, and thrombocytopenia. Clinicians who attempt to treat patients with large numbers of circulating tumor cells should consider modification of the administration of rituximab, i.e. slower infusion, dose reductions, diluted concentration, and tumor lysis precautions.

Although a thorough examination of all the ongoing rituximab trials is beyond the scope of this review, a few are worth mentioning. Treatment of residual microscopic disease provides the rationale for studies evaluating the adjuvant delivery of rituximab. The Eastern Cooperative Oncology Group is currently examining the adjuvant use of rituximab in two large randomized studies of indolent and aggressive B-cell lymphomas. Studies evaluating rituximab as consolidative therapy following high-dose chemotherapy with peripheral stem cell transplantation are ongoing. Studies investigating the augmentation of rituximab's antitumor effects with biologic therapies are being conducted with interferon-α, interleukin-2, granulocyte colony-stimulating factor, and granulocyte–macrophage colony-stimulating factor. At present, rituximab can be recommended for the treatment of relapsed indolent lymphoma, particularly in those patients with low tumor burdens. Patients may be considered for re-treatment with rituximab when the initial response exceeds six months. Rituximab treatment in patients with aggressive B-cell lymphoma who have either relapsed following transplantation or who are not suitable transplant candidates may also be considered. A number of interesting clinical trials in progress should determine the optimal use of rituximab, and participation is encouraged, rather than ad hoc treatment based upon small phase II experience.

CAMPATH-1H

CAMPATH-1H is a human immunoglobulin anti-CD52 MoAb that binds to the majority of all human lymphocytes and to most B-cell and T-cell lymphomas. CAMPATH-1H is administered as a two-hour infusion three times a week for a maximum period of 12 weeks. The starting dose is escalated based on the patient's tolerance to a maximum of 30 mg. CAMPATH-1H seems to have preferential activity on tumor cells residing in the bone marrow or circulating in the peripheral blood compared with those in the lymph nodes or extranodal sites. This clinical observation was confirmed in a phase II study in which 50 patients with relapsed indolent NHL were treated for 12 weeks.[35] Only 6 patients (14%) achieved a partial response, although there was a 50% response rate (4/8) in mycosis fungoides. CAMPATH-1H may have a more valuable role to play in the treatment of chronic lymphocytic leukemia (CLL) or T-cell prolymphocytic leukemia (T-PLL) owing to their respective predilections for the peripheral blood and bone marrow compartments. Treatment of 15 patients with T-PLL resulted in an impressive overall response rate of 73%;[36] however, all patients ultimately relapsed. A phase II study in 29 patients with relapsed CLL treated with CAMPATH-1H showed a 42% overall response rate, with a 12-month median duration of response.[37] Patients treated with CAMPATH-1H may experience significant infusion-related events, cytopenias, and infections secondary to neutropenia. Further investigation of its use for T-PLL or CLL will be required to define its optimal use.

RADIOLABELED ANTIBODIES

Despite the significant clinical activity of unconjugated MoAbs, the majority of patients with relapsed indolent lymphoma either fail to respond completely or ultimately relapse after response. Radionuclides have been conjugated to MoAbs in an effort to improve the response rate and duration of response (Table 13.2). The advantages of this approach include the observation that the lymphoid malignancies are exquisitely sensitive to radiation.[38] Further, tumor

Table 13.2 Experience with radioimmunoconjugates in B-cell lymphoma

Therapy	Radionuclide	ORR[a] (%)	Toxicity	Considerations	Refs
Tositumomab	Iodine-131 (^{131}I)	65–81 (17–38)	Myelosuppression Increased HAMA Secondary leukemia	Excellent response rate in unfavorable patients. Patients had <25% bone marrow involvement	39, 43
Tositumomab with stem cell support	Iodine-131 (^{131}I)	81 PFS 51 at 4 years	Myelosuppression Other organ toxicity	Cardiac and pulmonary dose-limiting toxicities	46
Ibritumomab	Yttrium-90 (^{90}Y)	82 (26)	Myelosuppression	Lower response rate in bulky disease; splenomegaly. Patients had <25% bone marrow involvement. Indium-111 required for imaging	40

[a]Overall response rate (complete response rate in parentheses); PFS, progression free survival.

cell death may be achieved either from direct emission of radioactive particles into cells that express the targeted antigen or as 'crossfire' in 'bystander' cells that fail to express the target antigen.[39] Finally, radioimmunoconjugates remain active in the setting of defective immune effector function.

Radionuclide properties

Radionuclides damage DNA primarily through the emission of β-particles,[40] which vary in energy and path length. To date, iodine-131 (^{131}I), which is relatively inexpensive and commercially available, is the most extensively used radionuclide, emitting both β-particles and γ-rays. The advantage of γ-emissions is the ability to perform localization and dosimetry studies; however, γ-particles also increase the radiation risk to family members and health care personnel; consequently patients receiving ^{131}I may require inpatient administration. The Nuclear Regulatory Commission revised their regulations for the release of patients administered ^{131}I therapy, and ultimately ^{131}I-based therapy may be conducted on an outpatient basis.[41] Yttrium-90 (^{90}Y) a pure β-emitter that can be delivered safely on an outpatient basis, releases higher-energy β-particles (2.3 MeV versus 0.61 MeV) that have a significantly longer path length (5–10 mm versus 0.8 mm). Hypothetically, bulky or poorly vascular tumor masses may respond more readily to ^{90}Y.

Administration and toxicity

In order to optimize biodistribution and deliver the radioimmunoconjugate to the lymph nodes and extranodal tumor sites, unlabeled antibody is initially infused to bind the $CD20^+$ cells present in the blood and spleen. Thus far, murine MoAbs have served as the delivery vehicles of the radionuclide owing to the longer half-life of chimeric antibodies and the resultant extended radiation exposure. While patients experience fewer infusion-related side-effects, murine antibodies are limited by the development of HAMA and the reduced ability to recruit human immune effector mechanisms. Ultimately, the prolonged half-life of chimeric antibodies may be alleviated by using a radionuclide with a short half-life or by re-engineering a chimeric antibody with a shorter serum half-life. The dose-limiting toxicity of radioimmunotherapy is predominantly myelosuppression, with a nadir typically between 5 and 7 weeks, with normalization of the blood counts by 12 weeks. The degree of cytopenia correlates with the dose of the radionuclide, prior chemotherapy, or radiation exposure, and the extent of bone marrow involvement prior to treatment.

Radioimmunotherapy clinical trials

To date, impressive response rates have been achieved with radioimmuno-conjugates in the treatment of NHL.[42–45] The most extensively tested radioimmunoconjugate is the ^{131}I-anti-B1 antibody (tositumomab, Bexxar), which recognizes and binds to the CD20 antigen. Phase I/II studies of tositumomab in relapsed but transplant-naive patients with B-cell NHL showed the maximally tolerated dose to be 75 cGy[42] and an overall response rate of 71% (with a 34% complete response rate). The dose-limiting toxicity was hematologic, and 15% patients developed HAMA. The multicenter pivotal trial with tositumomab included an unfavorable subset of patients who had received two or more prior therapies. Forty-four percent of patients had elevated lactate dehydrogenase (LDH) and 65% had disease larger than 5 cm. The overall response rate was 65% (with a 17% complete response rate), with a median duration of response of 6.5 months.[46] Kaminski et al[47] also tested tositumomab as primary therapy in newly diagnosed low-grade NHL, and found an overall response rate of 100%, but the development of HAMA was 31%.

Tositumomab has also been delivered at myeloablative doses followed by autologous stem cell support.[48] Twenty-nine patients with multiply recurrent low-grade or transformed NHL achieved a 79% complete response rate. Over a median follow-up time of 42 months, the overall survival rate was 68% and the progression-free survival rate was 42%. In an attempt to improve the duration of remissions, Press and colleagues[49] delivered tositumomab in combination with high-dose chemotherapy and autologous stem cell transplantation to patients with relapsed B-cell NHL. The dose-limiting toxicities were primarily gastrointestinal and pulmonary, and initial experience suggests that delivery of 25 Gy to healthy organs is feasible. Over a median follow-up of 18 months, the progression-free survival rate was 78%.

To determine the activity of radioimmunotherapy in previous recipients of rituximab, Gregory et al[50] retrospectively observed whether tositumomab can be safely administered after prior treatment with rituximab. Twenty-eight patients received therapeutic doses of tositumomab without discontinuation of the infusion, including one patient who was HAMA-positive at study entry. An ongoing prospective phase II multicenter trial is currently establishing the efficacy of this maneuver.

^{90}Y-2B8 (ibritumomab, Zevalin) is a radioimmunoconjugate composed of the murine G1 κ anti-CD20 monoclonal antibody (2B8), the linker chelator isothiocyanatobenzyl-MX-DTPA, and the radionuclide ^{90}Y. Because of the pure β-emission and consequent inability to undergo dosimetry, dosing is based on the body surface area of the patient, and patients are pretreated with indium-111 to ensure localization. Phase I/II studies[43] of ibritumomab determined the optimal dose of pretreatment rituximab to be 250 mg/m^2 and the ^{90}Y maximum tolerated dose to be 0.4 mCi/kg. The overall response rate was 67% in patients with indolent or intermediate-grade lymphoma, although an overall response rate of 82% was achieved in patients with low-grade lymphoma. The dose-limiting toxicity was hematologic, HAMA developed in only 2%, and the median time to progression was 12.9 months. The lower HAMA rate with ibritumomab compared with tositumomab may be attributed to pretreatment exposure to the chimeric antibody, rituximab, as opposed to the murine antibody, anti-B1.

Additional radioimmunoconjugates include the Lym-1 antibody (HLA-DR) and the LL2 antibody (CD22). DeNardo and colleagues[51] treated 20 relapsed NHL patients with ^{131}I-Lym-1 antibody given in fractionated doses in a phase I/II dose-escalation study. Only 29% of patients were able to receive the four planned treatments, primarily owing to hematologic toxicity. The overall response rate was 52% and the maximum tolerated dose was determined to be 100 mCi/m^2. Treatment with ^{131}I-LL2 antibody resulted in an overall response rate of 33%; however, owing to hematologic toxicity, five patients required stem cell infusion. Clinical trials are ongoing to determine to optimal treatment of the radiolabeled Lym-1 and LL2 antibodies.

The higher overall and complete response rates achieved with radio-immunoconjugates compared with unconjugated MoAbs must be weighed against their greater toxicity. The observed secondary leukemias after non-myeloablative and myeloablative doses of tositumomab and the delayed myelo-suppression are marrow toxicities of concern. Although the occurrence of leukemia has been observed among patients previously treated with multiple courses of alkylating agents, it suggests that some thought must be given to the design of treatment regimens using radioimmunoconjugates in combination with chemotherapy.

IMMUNOTOXINS

The conjugation of a toxin to a monoclonal antibody is an alternative approach to delivering an otherwise non-specific toxic therapy. Immunotoxins require internalization of the antigen-antibody complex whereby the toxin exerts its effects. Ricin, the most commonly used toxin, is a heterodimer that contains an A chain, which inhibits protein synthesis by inactivating the 60S ribosomal subunit of eucaryotic ribosomes, and a B chain, which regulates the transloca-tion of the toxin into the cell. Other toxins used include diptheria toxin, *Pseudomonas* exotoxin, and saporin.

Both the CD19 (anti-B4bR and HD37–dgA) and CD22 (IgG–RFB4–dgA) antigens have been targeted by ricin-based immunotoxins.[52–54] Response rates in patients with relapsed NHL have ranged from 5% to 20%, with profound toxicities including capillary leak syndrome, hepatitis, and thrombocytopenia. In an effort to circumvent the toxicity observed in patients with bulky tumors, anti-B4bR has also been tested following autologous transplant in the setting of minimal disease.[55] However, anti-B4bR failed to show any improvement in relapse-free or overall survival.

Several immunotoxins, varying in the antibody structure and toxin used, have been targeted to the CD25 antigen. DAB389IL-2 is a fusion toxin with moderate activity in patients with multiply recurrent mycosis fungoides, and has been FDA-approved. RFT5.dgA, an anti-CD25 antibody, linked to a degly-cosylated ricin A chain, has been tested in patients with relapsed Hodgkin's disease.[56] The majority of patients developed HAMA, and there were only two partial responses. The recombinant immunotoxin LMB-2 (anti-Tac(Fv)–PE38) targets CD25$^+$ cells and is composed of the Fv portion of the anti-Tac antibody and a truncated form of *Pseudomonas* exotoxin A. Four patients with refractory hairy cell leukemia showed clinically objective responses, with one patient remaining in complete remission after 11 months.[57] Because clinical trials show only modest activity and significant immunogenicity, the use of these immunotoxins is currently limited.

FUTURE CONSIDERATIONS

MoAbs have clinically significant activity in the lymphoid malignancies, and have become an integral component of the treatment armamentarium. Currently, direct comparisons of survival and response data between different antibody studies is confounded by differences in patient characteristics and enrollment criteria. Other unconjugated MoAbs currently under investigation include those targeted against the CD19, CD22, and HLA-DR antigens. Future targeted antigens include CD3 (a T-cell antigen) and CD30 (expressed in Hodgkin's disease and anaplastic large cell lymphomas). As the rapidly expanding availability of novel engineered antibodies for the lymphoid malignancies continues, careful design of prospective trials will need to be performed to accurately interpret clinical results.

REFERENCES

1. Erlich P, On immunity with specific reference to cell life. *Proc R Soc Lond* 1900; 66. 424.

2. Kohler G, Milstein C, Continuous cultures of fused cells secreting antibody of predefined specificity. *Nature* 1975; 256: 495–7.

3. Miller RA, Maloney DG, Warnke R et al, Treatment of B-cell lymphoma with monoclonal anti-idiotype antibody. *N Engl J Med* 1982; 306: 517–22.

4. Nadler LM, Stashenko P, Hardy R et al, Serotherapy of a patient with a monoclonal antibody directed against a human lymphoma-associated antigen. *Cancer Res* 1980; 40: 3147–54.

5. Nadler LM, Takvorian T, Botnick L et al, Anti-B1 monoclonal antibody and complement treatment in autologous bone-marrow transplantation for relapsed B-cell non-Hodgkin's lymphoma. *Lancet* 1984; ii: 427–31.

6. Miller RA, Oseroff AR, Stratte PT et al, Monoclonal antibody therapeutic trials in seven patients with T-cell lymphoma. *Blood* 1983; 62: 988–95.

7. Miller RA, Levy R, Response of cutaneous T cell lymphoma to therapy with hybridoma monoclonal antibody. *Lancet* 1981; ii: 226–30.

8. Brown SL, Miller RA, Horning SJ et al, Treatment of B-cell lymphomas with anti-idiotype antibodies alone and in combination with alpha interferon. *Blood* 1989; 73: 651–61.

9. Maloney DG, Brown S, Czerwinski DK et al, Monoclonal anti-idiotype antibody therapy of B-cell lymphoma: the addition of a short course of chemotherapy does not interfere with the antitumor effect nor prevent the emergence of idiotype-negative variant cells. *Blood* 1992; 80: 1502–10.

10. Meeker T, Lowder J, Cleary ML et al,

Emergence of idiotype variants during treatment of B-cell lymphoma with anti-idiotype antibodies. *N Engl J Med* 1985; **312**: 1638–63.

11. Maloney DG, Grillo-Lopez AJ, Bodkin DJ et al, IDEC-C2B8: results of a phase I multiple-dose trial in patients with relapsed non-Hodgkin's lymphoma. *J Clin Oncol* 1997; **15**: 3266–74.

12. Shan D, Ledbetter JA, Press OW, Apoptosis of malignant human B cells by ligation of CD20 with monoclonal antibodies. *Blood* 1998; **91**: 1644–52.

13. Tedder TF, Engel P, CD20: a regulator of cell-cycle progression of B lymphocytes. *Immunol Today* 1994; **15**: 450–4.

14. Press OW, Appelbaum F, Ledbetter JA et al, Monoclonal antibody 1F5 (anti-CD20) serotherapy of human B cell lymphomas. *Blood* 1987; **69**: 584–91.

15. Reff ME, Carner K, Chambers KS et al, Depletion of B cells in vivo by a chimeric mouse human monoclonal antibody to CD20. *Blood* 1994; **83**: 435–45.

16. Maloney DG, Smith B, Appelbaum FR, The anti-tumor effect of monoclonal anti-CD20 antibody (mAb) therapy includes direct anti-proliferative activity and induction of apoptosis in CD20 positive non-Hodgkin's lymphoma (NHL) cell lines. *Blood* 1996; **88** (Suppl 1): A2535.

17. Maloney DG, Liles TM, Czerwinski DK et al, Phase I clinical trial using escalating single-dose infusion of chimeric anti-CD20 monoclonal antibody (IDEC-C2B8) in patients with recurrent B-cell lymphoma. *Blood* 1994; **84**: 2457–66.

18. Maloney DG, Grillo-Lopez AJ, White CA et al, IDEC-C2B8 (rituximab) anti-CD20 monoclonal antibody therapy in patients with relapsed low-grade non-Hodgkin's lymphoma. *Blood* 1997; **90**: 2188–95.

19. McLaughlin P, Grillo-Lopez AJ, Link BK et al, Rituximab chimeric anti-CD20 monoclonal antibody therapy for relapsed indolent lymphoma: half of patients respond to a four-dose treatment program. *J Clin Oncol* 1998; **16**: 2825–33.

20. Davis TA, Final report on the safety and efficacy of retreatment with rituximab for patients with non-Hodgkin's lymphoma. *Blood* 1999; **94** (Suppl 1): A385.

21. Piro LD, White CA, Grillo-Lopez AJ et al, Extended Rituximab (anti-CD20 monoclonal antibody) therapy for relapsed or refractory low-grade or follicular non-Hodgkin's lymphoma. *Ann Oncol* 1999; **10**: 655–61.

22. Davis TA, White CA, Grillo-Lopez AJ et al, Single-agent monoclonal antibody efficacy in bulky non-Hodgkin's lymphoma: results of a phase II trial of rituximab. *J Clin Oncol* 1999; **17**: 1851–7.

23. Solal-Celigny P, Salles G, Brousse N et al, Rituximab as first-line treatment of patients with follicular lymphoma and a low-burden tumor: clinical and molecular evaluation. *Blood* 1999; **94** (Suppl 1): A2802.

24. Berinstein NL, Grillo-Lopez AJ, White CA et al, Association of serum Rituximab (IDEC-C2B8) concentration and anti-tumor response in the treatment of recurrent low-grade or follicular non-Hodgkin's lymphoma. *Ann Oncol* 1998; **9**: 995–1001.

25. Molica S, Levato D, Dattilo A et al, Clinico-prognostic relevance of quantitative immunophenotyping in B-cell chronic lymphocytic leukemia with emphasis on the expression of CD20 antigen and surface immunoglobulins. *Eur J Haematol* 1998; **60**: 47–52.

26. Foran JM, Rohatiner AZ, Cunningham D et al, European phase II study of rituximab (chimeric anti-CD20 monoclonal antibody) for patients with newly diagnosed mantle-cell lymphoma and previously treated mantle-cell lymphoma, immunocytoma, and small B-cell lymphocytic lymphoma. *J Clin Oncol* 2000; **18**: 317.

27. Coiffier B, Haioun C, Ketterer N et al, Rituximab (anti-CD20 monoclonal antibody) for the treatment of patients with relapsing or refractory aggressive lymphoma: a multicenter phase II study. *Blood* 1998; **92**: 1927–32.

28. Velasquez WS, Cabanillas F, Salvador P et al, Effective salvage therapy for lymphoma with cisplatin in combination with high-dose Ara-C and dexamethasone (DHAP). *Blood* 1988; **71**: 117–22.

29. Rodriguez MA, Cabanillas FC, Velasquez W et al, Results of a salvage treatment program for relapsing lymphoma: MINE consolidated with ESHAP. *J Clin Oncol* 1995; **13**: 1734–41.

30. Moskowitz CH, Bertino JR, Glassman JR et al, Ifosfamide, carboplatin, and etoposide: a highly effective cytoreduction and peripheral-blood progenitor-cell mobilization regimen for transplant-eligible patients with non-Hodgkin's lymphoma. *J Clin Oncol* 1999; **17**: 3776–85.

31. Vose JM, Link BK, Grossbard ML et al, Phase II study of rituximab in combination with CHOP chemotherapy in patients with previously untreated intermediate or high-grade non-Hodgkin's lymphoma. *Blood* 1999; **94**: A388.

32. Czuczman MS, Grillo-Lopez AJ, White CA et al, Treatment of patients with low-grade B-cell lymphoma with the combination of chimeric anti-CD20 monoclonal antibody and CHOP chemotherapy. *J Clin Oncol* 1999; **17**: 268–76.

33. Czuczman MS, Grillo-Lopez AJ, White CA et al, Rituximab/CHOP chemoimmunotherapy in patients with low grade lymphoma: progression free survival after three years follow-up. *Blood* 1999; **94**: A432.

34. Byrd JC, Waselenko JK, Maneatis TJ et al, Rituximab therapy in hematologic malignancy patients with circulating blood tumor cells: association with increased infusion-related side effects and rapid blood tumor clearance. *J Clin Oncol* 1999; **17**: 791–5.

35. Lundin J, Osterborg A, Brittinger G et al, CAMPATH-1H monoclonal antibody in therapy for previously treated low-grade non-Hodgkin's lymphomas: a phase II multicenter study. European Study Group of CAMPATH-1H Treatment in Low-Grade Non-Hodgkin's Lymphoma. *J Clin Oncol* 1998; **16**: 3257–63.

36. Pawson R, Dyer MJ, Barge R et al, Treatment of T-cell prolymphocytic leukemia with human CD52 antibody. *J Clin Oncol* 1997; **15**: 2667–72.

37. Osterborg A, Dyer MJ, Bunjes D et al, Phase II multicenter study of human CD52 antibody in previously treated chronic lymphocytic leukemia. European Study Group of CAMPATH-1H Treatment in Chronic Lymphocytic Leukemia. *J Clin Oncol* 1997; **15**: 1567–74.

38. Horning SJ, Natural history of and therapy for the indolent non-Hodgkin's lymphomas. *Semin Oncol* 1993; **20**: 75–88.

39. Nourigat C, Badger CC, Bernstein ID, Treatment of lymphoma with radiolabeled antibody: elimination of tumor cells lacking target antigen. *J Natl Cancer Inst* 1990; **82**: 47–50.

40. Simpkin DJ, Mackie TR, EGS4 Monte Carlo determination of the beta dose kernel in water. *Med Phys* 1990; **17**: 179–86.

41. Siegel JA, Revised Nuclear Regulatory Commission regulations for release of patients administered radioactive materials: outpatient iodine-131 anti-B1 therapy. *J Nucl Med* 1998; **39**: 28S–33S.

42. Kaminski MS, Zasadny KR, Francis IR et al, Iodine-131–anti-B1 radioimmunotherapy for B-cell lymphoma. *J Clin Oncol* 1996; **14**: 1974–81.

43. Witzig TE, White CA, Wiseman GA et al, Phase I/II trial of IDEC-Y2B8 radioimmunotherapy for treatment of relapsed or refractory CD20+ B-cell non-Hodgkin's lymphoma. *J Clin Oncol* 1999; **17**: 3793–803.

44. Knox SJ, Goris ML, Trisler K et al, Yttrium-90-labeled anti-CD20 monoclonal antibody therapy of recurrent B-cell lymphoma. *Clin Cancer Res* 1996; **2**: 457–70.

45. Press OW, Eary JF, Appelbaum FR et al, Phase II trial of ^{131}I-B1 (anti-CD20) antibody therapy with autologous stem cell transplantation for relapsed B cell lymphomas. *Lancet* 1995; **346**: 336–40.

46. Kaminski MS, Zelenetz AD, Press O et al, Multicenter phase III study of iodine-

131 tositumomab (anti-B1 antibody) for chemotherapy-refractory low-grade or transformed low-grade non-Hodgkin's lymphoma. *Blood* 1998; **92**: A1296.

47. Kaminski MS, Gribbin T, Estes J et al, I-131 anti-B1 antibody for previously untreated follicular lymphoma: clinical and molecular remissions. *Proc Am Soc Clin Oncol* 1998; **17**: A6.

48. Liu SY, Eary JF, Petersdorf SH et al, Follow-up of relapsed B-cell lymphoma patients treated with iodine-131-labeled anti-CD20 antibody and autologous stem-cell rescue. *J Clin Oncol* 1998; **16**: 3270–8.

49. Press O, Eary J, Liu S et al, A phase I/II trial of high dose iodine-131–anti-B1 monoclonal antibody, etoposide, cyclophosphamide, and autologous stem cell transplantation for patients with relapsed B-cell lymphomas. *Proc Am Soc Clin Oncol* 1998; **17**: A9.

50. Gregory SA, Leonard J, Coleman M et al, Bexxar can be safely administered in relapsed low-grade or transformed low-grade non-Hodgkin's lymphoma (NHL) patients after prior treatment with rituximab: initial experience for the expanded access study. *Blood* 1999; **94**: A396.

51. DeNardo GL, DeNardo SJ, Goldstein DS et al, Maximum-tolerated dose, toxicity, and efficacy of ^{131}I-Lym-1 antibody for fractionated radioimmunotherapy of non-Hodgkin's lymphoma. *J Clin Oncol* 1998; **16**: 3246–56.

52. Grossbard ML, Lambert JM, Goldmacher VS et al, Anti-B4-blocked ricin: a phase I trial of 7-day continuous infusion in patients with B-cell neoplasms. *J Clin Oncol* 1993; **11**: 726–37.

53. Stone MJ, Sausville EA, Fay JW et al, A phase I study of bolus versus continuous infusion of the anti-CD19 immunotoxin, IgG–HD37–dgA, in patients with B-cell lymphoma. *Blood* 1996; **88**: 1188–97.

54. Amlot PL, Stone MJ, Cunningham D et al, A phase I study of an anti-CD22–deglycosylated ricin A chain immunotoxin in the treatment of B-cell lymphomas resistant to conventional therapy. *Blood* 1993; **82**: 2624–33.

55. Grossbard ML, Multani PS, Freedman AS et al, A Phase II study of adjuvant therapy with anti-B4–blocked ricin after autologous bone marrow transplantation for patients with relapsed B-cell non-Hodgkin's lymphoma. *Clin Cancer Res* 1999; **5**: 2392–8.

56. Schnell R, Vitetta E, Schindler J et al, Treatment of refractory Hodgkin's lymphoma patients with an anti-CD25 ricin A-chain immunotoxin. *Leukemia* 2000; **14**: 129–35.

57. Kreitman RJ, Wilson WH, Robbins D et al, Responses in refractory hairy cell leukemia to a recombinant immunotoxin. *Blood* 1999; **94**: 3340–8.

Index